Gamification and Artificial Intelligence during COVID-19:
Case Studies in Health and Education

Carmen Bueno Muñoz /
Luis R. Murillo Zamorano /
José Ángel López Sánchez

Gamification and Artificial Intelligence during COVID-19: Case Studies in Health and Education

PETER LANG

**Bibliographic Information published by the
Deutsche Nationalbibliothek**
The Deutsche Nationalbibliothek lists this publication in the Deutsche
Nationalbibliografie; detailed bibliographic data is available online at
http://dnb.d-nb.de.

Library of Congress Cataloging-in-Publication Data
A CIP catalog record for this book has been applied for
at the Library of Congress.

Project co-financed by the European Regional Development Fund (80%)
and the Regional Government of Extremadura (file GR18123) /
Proyecto cofinanciado por el Fondo Europeo de Desarrollo Regional (80%)
y la Junta de Extremadura (expediente GR18123).

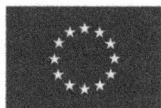

Unión Europea

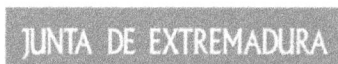

JUNTA DE EXTREMADURA

Consejería de Economía, Ciencia y Agenda Digital

Cover illustration: "hand with lighting" obtained from
© serazetdinov/istockphoto.com

ISBN 978-3-631-86987-1 (Print) · E-ISBN 978-3-631-87042-6 (E-PDF)
E-ISBN 978-3-631-87043-3 (EPUB) · DOI 10.3726/b19256

© Peter Lang GmbH
Internationaler Verlag der Wissenschaften
Berlin 2022
All rights reserved.

Peter Lang – Berlin · Bern · Bruxelles · New York · Oxford · Warszawa · Wien

This publication has been peer reviewed.

www.peterlang.com

Abstract

The health emergency caused by COVID-19 has been a global challenge. During this period, it was necessary to quickly develop solutions that were able to cope with the pandemic and help mitigate the effects that the new coronavirus was causing in many sectors. This book analyzes how gamification and artificial intelligence (AI) have been used during the COVID-19 pandemic in two areas that have been particularly affected: health care and education. To this end, a review of the main applications of gamification and AI during this period is made. We also analyze four cases framed in health care and education in which both resources, gamification and AI, are combined and their usefulness in the context characterized by COVID-19 is analyzed. Finally, some of the ethical issues surrounding gamification and AI in this scenario are examined.

Keywords: gamification, artificial intelligence, COVID-19, health, education.

Table of contents

1. Introduction

Since COVID-19 was declared a global pandemic on March 11, 2020, by the Director General of the World Health Organization, Tedros Adhanom, an unprecedented crisis has been unleashed (World Health Organization, 2020). Measures put in place to curb the spread of the coronavirus, such as facility closures, social distancing and home confinement, have forced a large number of activities and processes to shift to digital platforms, accelerating the digital transformation of all sectors (Fletcher and Griffiths, 2020; Weil and Murugesan, 2020). Therefore, it is not surprising that many of the projects aimed at slowing the spread of COVID-19 and mitigating its effects have taken place through digital means. During the pandemic, mobile applications (apps) and online platforms have been used to find solutions to help people adapt to the new circumstances and speed up the return to normality.

One of the sectors that have been most affected by the novel coronavirus is health care. The pandemic has required scientists and doctors worldwide to work quickly to advance the knowledge about COVID-19 and discover effective drugs and vaccines. Thanks to digital media, research can be conducted more quickly by immediately connecting professionals from different parts of the world and facilitating knowledge sharing (Cho et al., 2020; Masuda et al., 2021).

The pandemic has also posed a challenge to health systems. Hospitals have become overcrowded, and consequently, the quality of care for patients with other pathologies has decreased (Kretchy et al., 2021; Legido-Quigley et al., 2020). In this context, offering digital health care services can alleviate the burden on health care professionals and improve the quality of face-to-face care for patients in health care centers (Willems et al., 2021).

Another sector that has been directly affected by COVID-19 and, more precisely, by the measures to contain the spread of the virus, is education. Most educational institutions worldwide closed their doors during the onset of the pandemic, affecting more than 1.5 billion students (UNESCO, 2020), which has forced the adoption of methodologies based on digital media to conduct the teaching-learning process virtually.

This book addresses the use of two resources within the applications and digital platforms used during the pandemic in the aforementioned sectors: gamification and artificial intelligence (AI). Gamification is a design technique that seeks to *enhance* systems and create more engaging experiences that resemble those provided by games (Hassan and Hamari, 2020; Zainuddin et al., 2020). Gamification aims to motivate individuals and encourage them to engage in certain behavior (Feng et al., 2020; Kalogiannakis et al., 2021; Putz et al., 2020). This technique is growing, and two of its main areas of application are health care and education (Klock et al., 2020; Koivisto and Hamari, 2019; Swacha, 2021; Trinidad et al., 2021).

AI refers to the ability of machines to perceive, understand, make decisions, act and comprehend (Fosso Wamba et al., 2021; Mondal, 2020). AI is present in our daily lives through voice assistants, chatbots, and multiplatform content and product recommendation systems. AI has already been employed in the fight against previous viruses such as SARS-CoV-1 and MERS-CoV and holds great potential to help combat COVID-19 (Bansal et al., 2020).

Given this context, this book aims to analyze the use of gamification and AI in the health and educational fields during the pandemic. Thus, a review of the main applications of gamification and AI during this period is carried out, as well as an analysis of four cases in which gamification and AI are combined and their usefulness in the context of COVID-19 is characterized and examines some of the ethical issues surrounding gamification and IA during this period.

This book is structured as follows. After this introduction, which corresponds to Chapter 1, Chapter 2 focuses on the use of gamification during the period characterized by the new coronavirus. More precisely, the main applications of gamification in the context of COVID-19 in the health and educational fields are studied, as well as other relevant applications in sectors other than those previously mentioned. Chapter 3 focuses in a similar way on the use of AI, mainly in the health and educational fields.

Chapter 4 examines the application of gamification and AI during the pandemic through the study of four case studies. Two of these cases, DreamLab: Corona-AI and uMore, are framed in the health care environment, while two, Century and ELSA Speak, are in the educational field.

Specifically, DreamLab: Corona-AI is an investigation into the potential effect of molecules present in food and drugs on the disease caused by the new coronavirus, which uses gamification, AI and distributed computing. uMore is a mental health app created during the pandemic to help manage anxiety and stress during COVID-19. uMore is based on AI to offer personalized recommendations to its users and encourages the use of the app through gamification.

Century is a gamified educational platform that combines learning science, AI and neuroscience and has provided free access to its services to support teachers and students in this period of uncertainty. ELSA Speak is a gamified app aimed at individuals whose native language is not English. ELSA Speak uses speech recognition to detect and correct pronunciation errors made by the user. Chapter 4 discusses the role that these four apps have played during the pandemic and how gamification and AI are combined in them.

Chapter 5 discusses some of the ethical issues affecting gamification and IA in the context of the pandemic. Finally, Chapter 6 presents the conclusions and final reflections reached through writing this book.

2. Gamification during the COVID-19 crisis

2.1. Introduction

Gamification is a design technique that uses game-like elements to create motivating experiences (Feng et al., 2020; Putz et al., 2020). The game elements used in this technique do not form a closed list. Among the most recurrent are those that form the so-called PLB triad: *points, badges* and *leaderboards* (Leitão et al., 2021). Other examples are narrative, *feedback*, quests and progress bars. All these elements create a design that can reward users' behavior, surprise them and encourage collaboration or competition between several members (Schöbel et al., 2020). Regardless of the elements used, gamification aims to *enhance* systems and create more engaging experiences that resemble those provided by games (Hassan and Hamari, 2020; Zainuddin et al., 2020). It is often used to improve the motivation, performance and *engagement* of individuals (Trinidad et al., 2021).

Gamification is a booming technique whose use has spread to numerous fields, from marketing to *e-government* platforms (Contreras-Espinosa and Blanco, 2021; Whittaker et al., 2021). Among them, the most important field of application is education (Klock et al., 2020; Koivisto and Hamari, 2019). Studies point out that gamification motivates students and improves their learning outcomes (Kalogiannakis et al., 2021). Therefore, its use continues to increase over time in this field (Swacha, 2021). Likewise, in recent years, there has been a growing interest in gamification in the health care sector. In this context, gamification is used to promote healthy habits and behaviors such as physical exercise and to encourage self-management of different aspects related to health status (Trinidad et al., 2021).

The COVID-19 pandemic has been a global challenge. Governments have had to make decisions quickly to try to contain the spread of the virus and implement effective measures. In this context, public trust and cooperation are essential to achieve the desired goals (Devine et al., 2021). To this end, gamification can be used to encourage the adoption of behaviors that reduce the spread of COVID-19. Raab et al. (2021) detect the spontaneous appearance of gamification elements in the context of the pandemic. From these, they propose giving meaning to these elements and shaping the mechanics, dynamics and aesthetics through what they call "*strategic gamification*" of COVID-19 to encourage cognitive and emotional responses from the population. The elements of gamification that emerged spontaneously during the pandemic and the design patterns that Raab et al. (2021) attribute to each are as follows:

• *Points*: These authors point out that the figures for the number of people infected and the number of deaths from coronavirus, the number of tests and the number of vaccinations, among others, are similar to the points in a gamified design. In addition, they point out that the databases that collect this information are constantly updated and are usually visible on news websites, giving a ubiquitous character to these figures that quantify the magnitude of the pandemic.

• *Leaderboards*: These point-like figures serve as a basis for ranking the incidence of COVID-19 and the actions of governments in different cities, regions and countries. These *leaderboards* can create a picture of competition in which the locations with the lowest number of infected are the winners. Raab et al. (2021) advocate introducing other indicators, such as the number of hours spent by volunteers and monetary donations, to fight the pandemic to give recognition to those who dedicate the most effort to this cause.

• *Roles*: Although the use of masks and vaccinations are key factors in the strategy against the pandemic, they are met with reluctance by part of the population. Those who wear masks and get vaccinated play a very important role in the context of COVID-19. Raab et al. (2021) point out that masks can be seen as a sign of carrying out a responsible role that, in addition, confers certain advantages to the individual, such as the possibility of accessing certain places, for example shops and other establishments.

• *Collecting Resources*: At the beginning of the pandemic, not knowing how long the confinement would last and what the consequences would be, the population bought and stockpiled basic necessities such as canned food and toilet paper. In this context, problems arise when a certain percentage of individuals hoard resources; when individuals made excessive purchases, it is difficult for others to acquire the minimum necessary. Raab et al. (2021) point out that this hoarding behavior may be a means used by some individuals to maintain self-efficacy in complex situations, such as this health crisis. Thus, these authors propose using narratives to raise public awareness about the sensible distribution of resources and to enable individuals themselves to determine the appropriate level of stockpiling.

- *Archetypes*: Two of the main archetypes of games are heroes and villains. In the context of the pandemic, both are present. The heroes are represented, among others, by the health professionals who fight against the coronavirus, and the villains could be those who deny the existence of the virus. Raab et al. (2021) highlight the emergence of another type of hero: the famous COVID-19 infected. The announcement of having this disease by celebrities seems to be an effective tool to raise awareness of the pandemic. Positively perceived celebrities are portrayed as heroes who survive the disease. This narrative can make it easier for those individuals who distrust science and the media to become more aware of the pandemic and, therefore, to modify their behavior to try to avoid contagion.
- *Location-Based Gaming*: as a measure to contain the pandemic, location-based mobile applications have been developed, such as those that show the places with the highest incidence of COVID-19 or those that warn users if they are in a place at the same time as another person who has received a positive diagnosis of coronavirus. Raab et al. (2021) propose adding other functionalities to these location-based applications, such as pointing out which nearby entertainment venues are less crowded to avoid large gatherings of people.

The analysis of the spontaneous emergence of gamification and its proposal of "*strategic gamification*" to fight the pandemic serves as an introduction to analyze how this design technique has been used during this period. Specifically, this chapter studies the main applications of gamification in the context of COVID-19 in the health and education sectors, two of the most important areas in which this technique is used, as well as other relevant applications in other sectors.

2.2. Areas of application during COVID-19

2.2.1. Health

The pandemic has posed a challenge to health systems. Hospitals have become overcrowded, and as a consequence, the quality of care for patients with other pathologies has decreased (Kretchy et al., 2021; Legido-Quigley et al., 2020). In this context, offering a digital health service can alleviate the burden on professionals who practice in person and facilitate the provision of quality care to patients in health centers (Willems et al., 2021).

COVID-19 has led to the development of mobile health applications (apps) aimed at combating the effects of the new coronavirus (Singh et al., 2020). Citizens, health professionals and pandemic management authorities can all benefit from health apps during this period (Kondylakis et al., 2020). Apps are viewed as valuable tools for citizens, health professionals and decision-makers to address critical challenges posed by the pandemic, such as reducing the burden on hospitals, accessing reliable information, monitoring people's symptoms and mental health, and discovering new predictors.

According to the study by Almalki and Giannicchi (2021), two-thirds (66.95 %) of health apps related to COVID-19 have been created by governments or other authorities responsible for pandemic management. The next most important developer of health apps during this period was businesses (21.73 %). In contrast, few apps have been developed by non-profit organizations, hospitals or universities; fewer than 5 % of the total number of apps have been designed by these types of institutions.

Park et al. (2021) analyze which types of health apps are considered most needed by the population in the context of COVID-19. According to their study carried out in South Korea, the categories most frequently mentioned by the participants were *epidemiological investigation apps* (61.8 %), *self-management apps for self-isolation* (53.4 %), *self-route management apps* (52.7 %), *COVID-19 symptom management apps* (42.1 %), *COVID-19-related information provision apps* (29.5 %), *and mental health management apps* (23.5 %). In contrast, the main purpose of the health apps developed during the pandemic has been contact tracing and symptom tracking (Singh et al., 2020).

In any case, for these apps to be effective, the population needs to use them. Motivation to use them, both in general and during COVID-19, can be achieved through different pathways. For example, according to the study by Park et al. (2021), individuals with an underlying disease and those who have previously used a COVID-19–related app show a significantly greater intention to use a COVID-19–related health app than other individuals.

In this chapter, we focus on the study of gamification, a technique that can be effective in encouraging the participation of the population in health applications focused on the fight against COVID-19. Numerous empirical studies have been conducted before the pandemic about the application of gamification in the health care sector, and the results are positive (Koivisto and Hamari, 2019). This technique can be used to promote healthy habits that prevent or stop the progression of diseases or to increase the effectiveness of programs associated with health promotion (Lier and Breuer, 2019; Phillips et al., 2019).

2.2.1.1. Patient management

In the context of the pandemic, Marques et al. (2021) support using gamification to encourage the continued use of mental health apps to alleviate the adverse psychological effects caused by COVID-19. Seixas et al. (2021) advocate the use of gamification to facilitate chronic patients' use of new telemedicine applications that have emerged as a result of the pandemic. For example, Hsia et al. (2020) analyze the impact of a gamified mobile application dedicated to pediatric asthma patients and find that it improves their knowledge and control of the disease and reduces the number of visits to emergency rooms. Buheji (2020) points out that isolation during this period can accelerate cognitive decline in older adults due to the lack of interaction and communication with other individuals. Therefore, he proposes the use of gamification to mitigate memory loss among this group in the context of the pandemic. Araújo et al. (2021) suggest using gamification to monitor the health of this population group to prevent risks during periods of isolation.

Golden et al. (2021) developed an app to alleviate the impact of the pandemic on the mental health of health care professionals. This app has a gamified design that includes elements such as progress charts and personalized feedback. In addition, the authors of the app note that a future version should include badges to encourage greater participation.

However, according to Yoon et al. (2021), gamification could be viewed negatively in this context. Specifically, Yoon et al. (2021) analyze how *frontline health care workers* perceive psychological wellness apps. While a small percentage of the participants in this study considered that gamification provides entertainment, most of them believe that a gamified design based on points and badges that encourages competition can be demotivating and counterproductive. However, the *social influence* aspect was rated positively. Yoon et al. (2021) differentiate between gamification and *social influence*. However, *social influence* or *social pressure* is often considered in the literature as an element of gamification (e.g., Chou, 2019; Hamari and Koivisto 2015; Klock et al., 2020).

Social exposure could be key in gamified health apps. According to the study by Yang and Li (2021a), social interaction may positively affect user engagement in gamified health apps and make it easier for users to achieve their goals. Therefore, these authors recommend that app designers facilitate communication between users, especially with regard to complex achievements and the creation of large networks of contacts. In this way, exposure to the community is encouraged, exerting a motivating effect on its members. Interaction with other users offers other benefits, such as emotional support and the exchange of knowledge and experiences (Lin and Kishore, 2021).

2.2.1.2. Contact tracing

Contact tracing represents a fundamental strategy to stop the spread of infectious diseases. Thanks to current technology, contact tracing in the context of COVID-19 can be carried out through mobile applications that identify the physical proximity of users through GPS and Bluetooth on their *smartphones* (Osmanlliu et al., 2021). Examples of contact-tracking mobile applications are Immuni (www.immuni.italia.it) in Italy, STAYAWAY COVID (www.stayawaycovid.pt) in Portugal and Corona-Warn-App (www.coronawarn.app) in Germany. Gaining the adherence of a large volume of users represents a key factor for the performance of contact tracing applications (Colizza et al., 2021).

However, these applications, whose download and use are voluntary in most countries, have not received the expected level of acceptance by the authorities that developed them. The main reason for their low use can be found in the privacy concerns they generate (Williams et al., 2021; Zimmermann et al., 2021). The risk of giving away personal data does not seem to outweigh the potential benefits of these applications in curbing the pandemic (Zimmermann et al., 2021); thus, responsible authorities should devise strategies that encourage greater use of contact-tracking apps.

In the case of New Zealand, the Ministry of Health is responsible for NZ COVID Tracer, a mobile application that allows contact tracing through the use of Bluetooth technology and QR codes. Using Bluetooth, the app alerts users when it detects that they have been near another user who has tested positive for COVID-19. For QR codes, a user can scan these codes in public places, such as bars and restaurants, to create a record. When another user who has been to the same place at the same time is subsequently found to be infected, the app also alerts them (Ministry of Health of New Zealand, 2021).

On April 8, 2021, the New Zealand Ministry of Health updated NZ COVID Tracer to include some enhancements, including gamification (Dickinson, 2021). Following a gamified design, a log panel was enabled that made various indicators of application usage visible. This new, gamified version of the application provides users with data such as the total number of QR codes scanned, the number of active users, and the number of consecutive days each individual has used NZ COVID Tracer (Chen, 2021a; Dickinson, 2021). The aim of this gamified design is to encourage good habits and use of the app so that when individuals test positive for COVID-19, as much data as possible is available through the app to identify which people they have had contact with and, therefore, may have been infected (Chen, 2021a).

However, through gamification, participation in NZ COVID Tracer has not increased notably (Chen, 2021b). The factor that most seems to encourage the use of the app is the increase in the number of COVID-19 cases. If the perceived risk of contracting the disease increases, participation in NZ COVID Tracer increases. Conversely, when the volume of infections decreases, the number of active users of the app also decreases (Chen, 2021b).

2.2.1.3. Physical activity

Another negative health consequence of confinement is an increase in sedentary lifestyles. The activity level of the population has decreased in different countries during confinement (McCarthy et al., 2021; Yang and Koenigstorfer, 2020). Yang and Koenigstorfer (2020) analyze the effect of mobile sports training apps on sedentary behavior and conclude that they can mitigate the increase in sedentary behavior caused by the pandemic. They add that apps with a gamified design could be particularly helpful in this context.

One of the most popular gamified fitness systems is Fitbit. Fitbit is a company that offers *wearables* that measure physical activity, such as smartwatches and bracelets. The count of calories burned, hours of sleep and minutes of activity, among other parameters, are visible through its gamified app (Fitbit, 2021). In May 2020, Fitbit announced the launch of a study to detect COVID-19 through sensors in its devices before symptoms began. Over the next two months, more than 100,000 Fitbit users voluntarily participated in the study, helping to identify nearly 50 % of COVID-19 cases one day before users reported symptom onset with 70 % specificity (Heneghan, 2020). In addition, several researchers have used Fitbit in their studies of the health effects of the pandemic (e.g., Jiwani et al., 2021; Rezaei and Grandner, 2021).

2.2.1.4. Training and awareness

Finally, within the health care field, gamification has also been used to disseminate information and promote the prevention of COVID-19 infections. For example, gamification has been used to create educational posters to prevent the transmission of the virus (Borzenkova et al., 2021) and for awareness campaigns about COVID-19; its ability to connect with the young population has been of special interest (Zain et al., 2021).

Suppan et al. (2020a) explain how they have designed a virtual course to teach prehospital staff how to protect themselves against coronavirus. According to these authors, one of the most significant challenges they face is the correct learning of the protocols for putting on and taking off personal protective equipment, given that the teaching is not done in person. To solve this problem and promote staff interaction, they use gamification.

In a later study, Suppan et al. (2020b) analyzed the effectiveness of this gamified course. Both this and the proportion of action guides improve staff skills regarding procedures for using protective equipment, but there are no significant differences between them. However, it should be noted that those who have received the training with a gamified design have maintained their level of self-confidence in their ability to use the equipment, while the confidence of staff who have not received the training has fallen.

In conclusion, gamification has been applied in different areas within the health care field to combat COVID-19. These include apps for monitoring other diseases, contact-tracking systems, physical activity apps and awareness campaigns. Gamification is a widely used technique to incentivize certain behaviors and has also been used in these times of health crises.

2.2.2. Education

One of the sectors that have been directly affected by the measures to contain the spread of the virus is education. Most educational institutions worldwide closed their doors during the beginning of the pandemic, affecting more than 1.5 billion students (UNESCO, 2020), which made it necessary to transform educational methodologies and transfer teaching and learning to the digital plane. Confinement and urgent adaptation to virtual teaching represent a challenge for teachers and educational institutions. On the one hand, the absence of technological skills, electronic devices, anticipation and teaching skills prevent teaching from continuing during this crisis, which requires the use of videoconferencing and online work (Reyna-Figueroa et al., 2020). On the other hand, teachers must create mechanisms that motivate students to achieve their engagement virtually (Hall and Border, 2020).

Adapting to digital learning is a challenge for both students and teachers. However, this can lead to innovations that improve education in the aftermath of the pandemic (Torda, 2020). According to Sahin and Yurdugül's study (2020), when the pandemic takes place in the digital context, learners demand entertaining environments supported by gamification. These results are in line with the present reality in the educational environment. Education is one of the main areas of application (Klock et al., 2020; Koivisto and

Hamari, 2019), and most gamified experiences take place through digital media (Kalogiannakis et al., 2021).

2.2.2.1. *Gamified experiences, the results and areas of knowledge*

Several authors have developed proposals for the effective use of gamification during pandemics. Fontana (2020) argues that the pandemic affects mental health and is an obstacle for students. He makes use of gamification to solve this problem, creating a quiz associated with a multiplayer game that allows students to interact, giving rise to a virtual community. Fontana contends that although it does not replace face-to-face classes, it helps to overcome the loss of community caused by confinement. Moreover, students report difficulties concentrating on their studies as a result of the stress associated with the pandemic, impairing their academic performance (Kecojevic et al., 2020). Gamification can be useful in encouraging them to engage despite the exceptional circumstances surrounding them. Alsamawi and Kurnaz (2021) also advocate the use of gamification to mitigate the anxiety and stress generated by the pandemic on teachers and students in schools.

Guckian et al. (2020) propose developing gamified experiences through escape games to foster collaborative learning and teamwork during confinement. O'Connell et al. (2020) apply gamification to the training of medical residents, developing a gamified experience, inspired by a television program, that takes place virtually through teleconferencing. The activity is divided into different phases. The first one, executed individually, consists of a training level based on the Kahoot application, which is very recurrent for gamification in the classroom. The following phases are carried out in teams. After that, the students completed a questionnaire about the experience. Most of them stated that they enjoyed carrying out the activity, that it increased their commitment and that they learned, thanks to the game. They also remarked that this format is better than traditional lessons.

The results of these experiences are positive. According to the review by Nieto-Escamez and Roldan-Tapia (2021), many studies reviewed by these authors reported improvements in learning or student motivation. Other studies found a low level of participation by students, which is associated with a decrease in intrinsic motivation as a consequence of the pandemic. Other benefits of these activities are the improvement of motivation, commitment and group cohesion (López-Belmonte et al., 2020). Following the online teaching experience during confinement, the university students who participated in Razami and Ibrahim's (2021) study reported that they prefer a hybrid teaching model that combines face-to-face and online classes. In addition, these students point to gamification and animations as better tools to foster their engagement with digital learning, placing them above other resources such as virtual reality, augmented reality, and simulations.

Regarding the areas of knowledge in which gamification has been used in this period of the pandemic, according to the review by Nieto-Escamez and Roldan-Tapia (2021), most of the gamified activities developed in secondary education and higher education during the pandemic have been carried out in the disciplines of science, technology, engineering and mathematics (STEM disciplines). These findings are consistent with those of Swacha (2021), who reviews the state of research on gamification in education since 2013. Swacha (2021) concludes that the area with the most studies in this regard is *computer science*. This author argues that the interest in gamification from *computer science* may be because the difficulty of this discipline requires strategies that encourage student engagement and motivation. He assigns the same argument to engineering and mathematics, two of the other two main academic fields that use gamification.

2.2.2.2. *Gamified educational platforms*

There are numerous platforms used for gamified educational experiences that are available to schools, teachers and students. These platforms are developed by different entities. For example, Solve Education! is a *nonprofit organization* from Singapore that aims to provide quality education to children and young people around the world who lack access to education. To achieve this goal, Solve Education! develops innovative technology based on gamification (Solve Education, 2021a). Their application provides personalized content and instant *feedback*, as well as allows students to carry out their learning in a flexible way (Solve Education, n.d.-a). In April 2020, they added new functionality focused on COVID-19 awareness based on verified information about the coronavirus to encourage preventive behaviors in a fun way (Solve Education, n.d.-b).

Solve Education! has played an important role in maintaining education during confinement by allowing students to continue learning in a motivating way using gamification. Lenovo, a Chinese multinational technology company, has decided to partner with the *nonprofit* Solve Education! and fund its initiatives so that children in countries such as Indonesia, Malaysia, Nigeria and Thailand can access quality education (Lenovo, 2021).

When a teacher decides to carry out a gamified experience with their students, they usually utilize the preexisting gamified platform Kahoot (Kalogiannakis et al., 2021). Kahoot is an educational platform that allows the creation of online quizzes and has a gamified design. Since its creation in 2013, more than *5 billion* individuals have participated in it, including half of the teachers and students in the U.S. in 2020 (Kahoot, 2021). Martín-Sómer et al. (2021) used Kahoot during the pandemic to counteract the loss of interest of university students caused by distance learning. Kalleny (2020) uses this platform in the last 10 minutes of class to review the content taught during the session. Banava et al. (2021) combine Kahoot and Zoom to continue teaching dental students virtually despite the restrictions arising from COVID-19.

Another gamified educational platform is Science Level Up, which focuses on teaching science to *elementary, middle*, and *high school students through a* gamified design that includes elements such as points and leaderboards. Park and Kim (2021) build on this platform to investigate the effects of gamification in the context of pandemics. The choice of Science Level Up to carry out their study is based on the fact that school students can access it through their computers and *smartphones* and, in addition, public schools in South Korea offer it free of charge to their students. As a result, they found that the use of this gamified platform has a positive impact on the motivation of students and facilitates the understanding of the course material.

In addition to using gamified platforms such as Kahoot and Science Level Up, teachers can create their own gamified experiences by designing them from scratch or developing gamified applications from available resources. The latter is the case of Areed et al. (2021), who created a gamified application using MIT App Inventor, an intuitive programming environment for creating apps for *smartphones* and *tablets*. MIT App Inventor is a free resource that permits creating apps in less than 30 minutes. Since its inception, more than six million users have registered, and nearly 30 million apps have been created (MIT App Inventor, 2021). Areed et al. (2021) use the MIT App Inventor to develop a gamified app through which university students take quizzes. They found that thanks to the gamified app, students' grades, critical thinking skills and autonomy in the learning process improved.

Another example of a gamified educational platform is the Gamified Educational Network (GEN), a website developed by *Ontario Tech University* in Canada that allows students to provide feedback to their peers through video assessments. During the pandemic, Guérard-Poirier et al. (2020) used the GEN to continue teaching surgical skills to medical students at the University of Montreal. Given its practical nature, if GEN had not been used, the surgical skills development of these students would have been disrupted by COVID-19.

In short, during the pandemic, schools, teachers and students have had access to different gamified alternatives capable of generating interest in students. As mentioned above, studies suggest that gamification has a positive effect on student motivation, facilitates their *engagement* with subjects, enables the acquisition of knowledge and, as a result, improves their final grades (López-Belmonte et al., 2020; Nieto-Escamez and Roldan-Tapia, 2021; O'Connell et al., 2020). This concept is key in the context of the pandemic. Measures to contain the virus have forced schools to shift teaching to the digital plane, and students' mental health and interest have suffered (Fontana, 2020; Kecojevic et al., 2020).

In this time of uncertainty, gamification appears to be an effective strategy to continue teaching and learning. Although no review has been found in this regard, it seems that teachers have maintained the trend of previous years and have resorted to preexisting gamified platforms instead of developing their own designs (Kalogiannakis et al., 2021). This issue may be due to the time and cost involved in the development of gamified systems, although, as mentioned, resources are currently available that facilitate this work, such as MIT App Inventor. In any case, COVID-19 has caused an unprecedented crisis that has required quick and effective solutions.

2.2.3. Other

In addition to education, there are other areas where gamification has been used during the pandemic. The spread of the coronavirus has forced companies to adapt to telecommuting and to close establishments that offer nonessential goods and services. Workers, without the supervision of their superiors, may devote less effort to their work. Gamification is a technique increasingly employed in this environment that can help prevent this (Spanellis et al., 2020). In the context of the pandemic, where measures implemented to prevent the spread of the coronavirus also hinder social relations, both companies and employees have shown an interest in the adoption of gamification (Tayal et al., 2020).

BBVA is a Spanish bank that has long offered training to its employees through its Campus BBVA platform, even before the pandemic. Campus BBVA compiles its content in different formats, such as videos, podcasts, simulators and game-based learning experiences. In addition, this e-learning platform has a recommendation system based on each employee's interests. During the pandemic, the hours of use of Campus BBVA increased dramatically; in the first 48 days of confinement, usage increased almost 450 % from the previous 48 days (Baeza, 2020).

Pilar Concejo, *the Global Head of Learning at BBVA*, points out that gamification is very important within the Campus BBVA platform, as it allows the creation of experiences that motivate employees, encourages their commitment and helps them advance continuously and sustainably over time (Baeza, 2021). BBVA is aware of how essential it is to train its employees and of the need to prepare them to face today's challenges. The COVID-19 pandemic has accelerated the transformation processes of many companies, and BBVA is no exception. To update and reinforce the key skills that employees must possess to drive the transformation and future of the bank, BBVA has launched The Camp, a gamified experience inspired by a mountain where employees progressively learn key skills (Baeza, 2021).

In addition to employee training, gamification can also be used in the business environment as a marketing tool. In the digital world, gamifying communities of users of a brand positively affect brand engagement, which in turn affects brand equity (Xi and Hamari, 2020). It can also influence customer behavior in e-commerce (Huseynov, 2020; Kamboj et al., 2020).

From this, companies have been able to benefit in order not to lose sales or brand image during confinement. In this period, interaction with potential customers was achieved through the internet in response to the closure of shops, and gamification represents an alternative to mitigate these adversities. In conclusion, gamification is a technique that has provided opportunities in the context of the pandemic both in health and education as well as in other sectors such as business.

Gamification has also been helpful in numerous projects and initiatives created to fight the effects of coronavirus through the collective efforts of citizens. According to the review by Kankanamge et al. (2020) on the use of this technique in times of crisis, gamification is used to encourage citizen participation in collaborative activities. Furthermore, they add that its popularization can lead to the establishment of a gamified culture. Here, monopolistic interfaces are transformed into spaces for exchange, which represents a great opportunity for managing crises such as the coronavirus. Moreover, Romano et al. (2021) analyze the effects of gamification in mobile applications that promote citizen participation and find that this technique improves the user experience and encourages their engagement, contributing to the success of this type of initiative.

3. Artificial intelligence during the COVID-19 crisis

3.1. Introduction

There is no generally accepted definition of AI (Naudé, 2021). Mondal (2020) offers a brief and concise definition: "*Artificial (made by human) intelligence (power of thinking) is the study of machines which can sense, make decision and act like human beings*" (Mondal, 2020, p. 390). The main capabilities that AI must possess are the ability to perceive, the ability to understand, the ability to act and the ability to learn. AI relies on different technologies, such as sensors, *machine learning* (ML), *deep learning* (DL), *natural language processing* (NLP), *computer vision* and *image recognition* (Fosso Wamba et al., 2021).

One of the most widespread terms among those mentioned above is ML, which is the ability of machines to "learn" (van Assen et al., 2020). To carry out this learning, understood as an improvement in its performance, the algorithm needs to be fed with data (Zhang and Lu, 2021). Additionally, a distinction is usually made between *supervised, semisupervised and unsupervised methods* of ML (Cichos et al., 2020).

DL is another term whose popularity has recently grown. DL, which can be considered a *subset* of ML, uses more complex algorithms. DL algorithms require considerably larger amounts of data and computational power than ML to provide accurate predictions (van Assen et al., 2020). A simple distinction between ML and DL is that ML makes predictions based on statistical methods and observed patterns, while DL relies on *multilayered statistical sequences* to identify patterns in patterns (Cope et al., 2020).

AI has already been employed to control previous viruses, such as SARS-CoV-1 and MERS-CoV (Bansal et al., 2020). With the emergence of COVID-19, AI has gained interest (Cossio and Gilardino, 2021). Some of the factors behind its expansion during the COVID-19 pandemic are the following (Coombs, 2020):

- *Consumer preferences changing to favor AI*: Social distancing as a measure to curb contagion has led to consumers preferring to use technologies that allow their experience to be self-managed. AI can reduce in-store interaction, for example, through contactless payment. The fear of contracting COVID-19 may help overcome some consumers' reluctance to use AI applications and encourage their use.
- *Increasing familiarity with AI technologies*: the need to use technology for teleworking or online teaching fosters familiarity with computing. The development of this computer culture in society may cause individuals to be more receptive to other technologies, such as AI-based technologies.
- *Increased business confidence in AI*: COVID-19 has led to an increase in teleworking to try to curb the expansion of the virus. Nevertheless, because certain tasks need to be carried out in person, such as cleaning, some companies have opted for AI-based robots to perform these in-person jobs and, in this way, protect employees from possible exposure to the virus. The pandemic has also accelerated the deployment of AI-based technology in companies that were in the development phase.

At the beginning of the pandemic, it was thought that AI would be able to curb the effects caused by the new coronavirus. From the very beginning, researchers specializing in the field of AI devoted their efforts to finding solutions to combat the crisis caused by COVID-19 (Raza, 2020). However, despite the potential of AI to combat the pandemic, its practical applications during this period have not lived up to its expectations. This issue has been mainly due to the scarcity of *datasets* (Naudé, 2020).

As mentioned above, the development of AI applications requires large datasets to train the algorithms and allow them to work properly, which is an obstacle in areas where the sensitivity level of the data is high and where the preservation of privacy is of great importance. In these cases, it is more complicated to create AI applications due to the lack of large datasets on which to base the learning of the algorithms. One of the most obvious fields where this occurs is health care.

According to the review by Abd-Alrazaq et al. (2020), the datasets used in the development of AI applications proposed as of April 2020 to combat COVID-19 are primarily from public databases such as the *National Center of Biotechnology Information* (NCBI, part of the U.S. National Library of Medicine), GitHub (an online repository for hosting projects and controlling code versions), and Kaggle (an online *data science* community). Other data sources used for AI development during the onset of the pandemic include those from medical centers and government sources such as the *Chinese Centers for Disease Control and Prevention.* To a lesser extent, data published in the literature and on news websites have also been used. Likewise, individuals have been recruited to participate in particular studies.

However, there are other *subsets* within AI that can be useful in the context of the pandemic and especially in health care. In 2017, Google presented a new approach to machine learning that, unlike traditional ML methods, does not require a large, centralized dataset but rather bases its training on multiple data sources distributed across multiple devices. They called this innovative approach *federated learning* (FL). FL generated little impact after its presentation. However, it has gained more prominence in recent years because of its ability to safeguard privacy and, as a consequence, its potential for use in health care (Hao, 2019).

In FL, the training of statistical models is carried out on remote devices, with the term device being generally understood to include *smartphones*, IoT devices, and even organizations (Li et al., 2020a). For example, in the health care sector, the ML process can take place in a decentralized way in each hospital; then, model features are transferred to train the algorithm and develop knowledge collaboratively. Under this FL approach, the privacy of patients is preserved, as their data remain within the hospital and training the algorithm with a large dataset is achieved if a sufficient number of health care institutions participate in the process (Rieke et al., 2020).

In the context of COVID-19, there is a need for collaboration between institutions and organizations from different countries to accelerate the development of solutions to the pandemic, including those related to health. In this scenario of international collaboration, LF can be very useful. For example, Dou et al. (2021) applied FL to generate an AI model to assess coronavirus disease from *chest computed tomographies* of patients. The exploration of algorithms using FL takes place in hospitals in various countries. In this way, the privacy of the patients is preserved, as the data are not transferred for centralized storage and use, which is of great importance, as the medical images of the patients represent sensitive material.

Thus, this chapter focuses on the study of the use of AI during the pandemic without specifying technical questions about the characteristics of the systems on which it is based. That is, no distinction is made between ML, DL and FL, among others. Specifically, this chapter analyses the different applications that have been developed based on AI in the health and educational fields, as well as outstanding applications in other sectors.

3.2. Areas of application of AI to COVID-19

3.2.1. Health

3.2.1.1. Prediction and monitoring

On December 31, 2019, seven days before scientists in China identified the virus and nine days before they notified the WHO, the company BlueDot warned its customers about the possibility of the onset of what appeared to be a new type of pneumonia (Allam, 2020; Long and Ehrenfeld, 2020). BlueDot also predicted the spread of the new coronavirus to Bangkok, Seoul, Taipei, and Tokyo within days of its appearance in Wuhan (Niiler, 2020). The question is, how could BlueDot have known about the evolution of COVID-19 in advance? The answer lies in AI.

BlueDot is a Canadian company that, through AI-based software, locates, tracks and predicts the spread of infectious diseases. Prior to COVID-19, BlueDot made accurate predictions about the spread of H1N1 in 2009, Ebola in 2014 and Zika in 2016 (Allam et al., 2020). To do this, it analyses data 24 hours a day. These data come from both official health sources, such as the *Centers for Disease Control* and the WHO, and unofficial sources. Among the latter are those from which they obtain data about the weather, the movements of travelers on commercial flights and the human, animal and insect populations (BlueDot, n.d.; Bowles, 2020). Among these data are data on the movement of commercial air travelers, which were the basis for BlueDot's first scientific work on COVID-19 (BlueDot, n.d.). In their analysis, Bogoch et al. (2020), the founder and several employees of BlueDot, used data generated from the *International Air Transport Association* (IATA) to quantify the volume of passengers traveling from Wuhan and predicted 8 of the first 10 cities reached by COVID-19 (BlueDot, n.d.).

Metabiota is a U.S. company similar to BlueDot in that its mission is to estimate, mitigate and manage the risk of epidemics through AI (Metabiota, 2020). As BlueDot did, Metabiota made accurate predictions about the evolution of the spread of the new coronavirus. In particular, Thailand, South Korea, Japan and Taiwan were identified as the countries most at risk before cases were reported there (Heilweil, 2020). Metabiota also uses flight data to make its predictions through AI. In addition, this company is investigating the potential of information from *social media* to estimate the risk of the occurrence of an epidemic (Heilweil, 2020). Dr. Kamran Kahn, CEO of BlueDot, on the other hand, rejects the possible use of *social media data* for predictions because these data are *too messy* (Niiler, 2020).

Both cases, BlueDot and Microbiota, show the potential of AI to predict the evolution of the new coronavirus. During the early pandemic, several AI-based models were developed to predict parameters related to COVID-19. For example, Al-Qaness et al. (2020) created a model to predict the number of coronavirus cases in the next 10 days based on confirmed cases in the previous days. Mesgarpour et al. (2021) propose a model to predict the spread of COVID-19 in public transportation.

However, as Marabelli et al. (2021) argue, the use of AI to make predictions about the evolution of COVID-19 may cause inequalities and negatively affect certain minorities and vulnerable population groups with few resources. If algorithms make their predictions based on the number of hospitalized patients, they may give erroneous results in areas with a higher percentage of individuals without access to health care. In such a case, the algorithm misinterprets that the incidence of COVID-19 in the area is low, leading to inaccurate predictions and risk of discrimination against vulnerable populations.

Contact tracing is another potential application of AI in the context of the pandemic (Vaishya, 2020). However, according to the review by Abdulkareem and Petersen (2021), there is no evidence that the contact tracing applications that alert users if they have been near a confirmed COVID-19 case in the previous days for a certain period of time use AI. Among the apps they cite are COVIDSafe (Australia), Ketju (Finland), CoronaApp (Germany), StopCovid (France) and NZ COVID Tracer (New Zealand).

Another application of AI is social control, understood as monitoring compliance with measures to curb the spread of COVID-19, such as interpersonal distancing and the use of masks (Naudé, 2020). Health authorities in some countries, such as South Korea and China, have employed AI to monitor the movements of infected citizens and their contacts. This technology is based on algorithms that use data from security camera images, credit card payments, *social media* and *mobile* GPS, among others. In this way, the aim is to control the spread of the virus (Lin and Hou, 2020).

Moreover, according to the study by Mbunge et al. (2021), China is the leading country in the application of AI for the detection, diagnosis, surveillance and monitoring of COVID-19. These authors suggest that this may be due to the availability of COVID-19 data in China. In any case, to safeguard the rights of the population, public COVID-19 *digital surveillance* systems should be time-limited. That is, the period for which data will be collected, the purpose of the data collection and when the permissions will expire (Sekalala et al., 2020) should all be established.

Other AI-based proposals for social control during COVID-19 include the following. Tang et al. (2021) suggest employing a solution based on the union of AI and the previously proposed Bluetooth technology (see Tang et al., 2020) to create a contact-tracking system within health care facilities. The system of Tang et al. (2020, 2021) represents a fast and simple solution that protects the privacy of individuals and allows the detection of possible contagions indoors. Its application in health care facilities could help contain the spread of coronavirus in an environment where large numbers of COVID-19 patients are concentrated, decreasing the risk of other patients and health care staff contracting the disease and infecting more individuals. Karaman et al. (2021) developed an AI-based system to monitor the distance between individuals in public spaces from camera images that can be installed in public places. Barnawi et al. (2021) used AI to monitor potential cases of COVID-19 through aerial thermal imaging.

3.2.1.2. *Patient management*

Patient management is another area of health care where the use of AI during the pandemic has been raised. He et al. (2021) advocate the use of AI in the field of digital health in the context of COVID-19. Aware of the reluctance that the use of new technologies may raise among certain population groups, these authors advocate the development of applications based on AI to monitor the evolution of the disease in patients with mild symptoms. Patients with mild symptoms of COVID-19 infection tend to be young people who are also more receptive to the use of new technologies. Therefore, this segment of the population seems to be the most suitable for the introduction of AI as a disease surveillance tool. He et al. (2021) propose the development of AI-based mobile applications in the following three domains to improve the experience of COVID-19 patients living with the disease at home:

- Provide reliable information about COVID-19, the areas of greatest risk and the symptoms it can produce: through AI, the information offered to each user could be personalized by analyzing their search history or the area in which the individual is located.
- Tracking the health status of each COVID-19 patient: AI could analyze an individual's symptoms and physical condition through text and voice messages. The results would determine each patient's diagnosis and treatment, and personalized recommendations and advice could be provided.
- Community support: AI could detect the health and emotional state of patients and, with their consent, share this information with their loved ones. Forums could also be created in which to share the experience with the community, control the content that is published and help other patients.

These proposals by He et al. (2021) are aimed at the use of AI via *smartphones*. Jadczyk et al. (2021) advocate using specific AI-based technology to monitor the evolution of COVID-19 patients: voice assistants. Voice assistants and, in particular, smart speakers have gained popularity in recent years. They are increasingly found inside homes (Mishra et al., 2021). Jadczyk et al. (2021) highlight the importance of voice assistants for the presence and future of telemedicine. In the context of COVID-19, voice assistants can be useful to remotely perform triage, diagnosis and assessment during the course of patients' illness, which avoids face-to-face interaction between doctors and patients at a time when personal protective equipment (PPE) is in short supply. PPE is essential to prevent health care professionals from being infected by the coronavirus. In the absence of PPE, voice assistants can be useful for assessing the condition of patients, making diagnoses and deciding on treatments remotely.

Amazon is one of the leading developers of voice assistants. During the pandemic, Amazon directed its efforts to make Alexa, its virtual assistant, helpful to its users. To do so, they have enabled the option to check for symptoms related to COVID-19 and the risk of contracting the disease in countries such as Canada, Mexico, the United States, Japan and India. Users simply ask "Alexa, what can I do if I think I have coronavirus?" and Alexa asks them a series of questions. The user's answers are then evaluated, and based on guidance from the health authorities in the country in question, information is provided (Amazon, 2020).

Another application of AI is through *chatbots*, which are computer programs that simulate human language and are able to dialog with individuals through AI (Huang and Chueh, 2021; Roy and Naidoo, 2021). During the pandemic, the number of consultations made to health care professionals have increased dramatically. Call centers have limited resources, mainly related to staffing and infrastructure. The high volume of calls has led to bottlenecks on telephone lines, making it difficult to provide quality information to patients and hampering the management and control of the virus (Ahuja et al., 2020). In this context, *chatbots* can be used to reduce call volume and facilitate communication with patients. They can provide guidance to patients who have tested positive for COVID-19, provide clinical information, and address questions raised by the public without overwhelming call centers (Ahuja et al., 2020).

Different governments have launched chatbots to answer citizens' questions about COVID-19. They are most commonly accessed through the WhatsApp application. To start a conversation, the user must save a certain phone number provided by the authorities that is linked to the chatbot and write the word "hello" in the language used in each country. After that, he can ask the questions he wants to resolve. Some governments that have created this type of chatbot are those of Spain (La Moncloa, 2020), the United Kingdom (GOV. UK, 2020) and India (Government of India, 2021). The WHO has also created a similar chatbot (WhatsApp, 2021).

Chatbots that are accessed through means other than the WhatsApp application, such as websites, have also been developed. This case is true for the chatbot developed by 1MillionBot, a Spanish entity focused on the creation of chatbots. 1MillionBot is part of the Spanish company IT&IS, which is dedicated to the development of different technological projects. Within the framework of the pandemic, 1MillionBot devised the chatbot Carina. Carina is equipped with AI and offers contrasting information in Spanish about more than 300 topics related to COVID-19. Some of the Carina answers included "what should I do if I have symptoms", "how many people are infected", "how many people have been cured", "what should I do if I have symptoms" and "what should I do if I live with an infected person"? Specifically, this AI-based chatbot is able to effectively answer 97.10 % of the questions asked (1MillionBot, 2021a). It is based on information obtained from the WHO, the Spanish Ministry of Health, the *Center for Disease, Control and Prevention* of the United States and scientific articles (TorreJuana, 2020).

Carina is available on the websites of more than 300 companies and institutions in countries such as Spain, Ecuador, Colombia, Chile, Mexico and the United States. Some examples of entities whose websites on which this chatbot has been inserted are national, regional and local government bodies, universities and the media (1MillionBot, 2021b). It should be noted that 1MillionBot has made Carina available to all public bodies that request it free of charge, as they consider it a contribution to society (TorreJuana, 2020).

The use of chatbots in the health field during the pandemic has not been limited to the resolution of doubts about the new coronavirus. For example, Wysa is a mobile application dedicated to mental health. It is an AI-based chatbot that helps its users manage anxiety and depression (Wysa, n.d.). The empirical study of the effectiveness of this app conducted by Inkster et al. (2018) reveals promising results as an aid in anxiety management.

During the pandemic, Wysa collaborated with experts from *Cincinnati Children's Hospital and the University of Cincinnati* to develop the COVID Anxiety app. This mobile app, like Wysa's app, consists of an AI-based chatbot. The goal of the COVID Anxiety app is to assist in the management of pandemic-associated anxiety through conversations and relaxation exercises. Among the methods this app uses to reduce stress for its users are cognitive behavioral therapy and visualization. Prior to launching the COVID Anxiety app, pretests were conducted. Specifically, initial versions of the app were presented to dozens of *Cincinnati Children's Hospital* patients who participated on a voluntary basis and who reported high levels of satisfaction with the app (Cincinnati Children's, 2020).

In any case, although chatbots can be useful to solve doubts and evaluate symptoms, it should be kept in mind that technology is not able to provide the human contact that certain patients need in this period where isolation has become more acute (Almalki and Giannicchi, 2021).

3.2.1.3. *Diagnosis and prognosis*

Another area of application of AI during the pandemic is in the diagnosis and prognosis of COVID-19 disease severity. Numerous studies have been conducted during this period on the ability of AI to analyze images, primarily chest radiographs, to diagnose COVID-19 and differentiate it from other types of pneumonia (e.g., Chrzan et al., 2021; Dorr et al., 2020; Salvatore et al., 2021), finding that AI can be very useful for this purpose. Reviews on the application of AI to the analysis of clinical images, such as X-rays and CT scans by Bouchareb et al. (2021) and Shaikh et al. (2021), conclude that AI has great potential to facilitate the diagnosis, monitoring and prognosis of COVID-19.

For example, Zhang et al. (2021a) found in their empirical study that the average diagnosis time by the AI-based diagnosis method they propose is less than the time required by the traditional diagnosis method (0.744 minutes by the AI-based method versus 3.623 minutes according to the traditional method). Furthermore, AI also improves the accuracy of the proposed method by Zhang et al. (2021a): the accuracy rate of the AI-based diagnostic method is 97.73 %, versus 83.72 % for the traditional method. That is, AI seems to improve both the diagnosis time and its accuracy rate, bringing a competitive advantage (Zhang et al., 2021a).

However, it should be noted that Marabelli et al. (2021) discuss the potential negative effects of AI-based solutions in the context of COVID-19. In the case of their application to disease diagnosis, the effectiveness of these algorithms depends on the *training data* entered beforehand, and certain ethnicities may be underrepresented in the datasets used. As a result, misdiagnosis can occur. Furthermore, this problem may become more serious if the use of this technology continues to expand.

The diagnosis of COVID-19 is not the only application of AI analysis of radiographs in the context of the pandemic. For example, Jiao et al. (2021) applied AI to the analysis of chest X-rays to predict the severity of COVID-19. According to their study, radiograph-based AI improves performance in predicting the risk of progression to critical status, which can help identify high-risk patients early and facilitate disease management. Other studies using AI to analyze *clinical images* to predict the severity of this disease include Chassagnon et al. (2021), Lassau et al. (2021), Li et al. (2020c), and Mushtaq et al. (2021). As in other applications, for AI to be useful in this area, large datasets must first be collected to train the algorithm, which usually consists of hundreds or thousands of images (Summers, 2021).

Other applications of AI to predict the severity of disease caused by the new coronavirus are through the analysis of *protein profiling* (Yaşar et al., 2021) and the analysis of individual factors such as gender, age and *health condition* (Li et al., 2020b). Through AI, it has also been detected that some demographic and clinical data of COVID-19 patients, such as their platelet count and leukocyte count, are factors through which mortality can be predicted (Zhang et al., 2021b). Additionally, AI has been used in other health care areas in COVID-19 patients, such as cardiology (Haleem et al., 2021) and ophthalmology (Hallak et al., 2020). In addition, the potential usefulness of AI for screening has been noted if other clinical manifestations, such as dermatological problems, are added (Sadoughifar et al., 2020).

3.2.1.4. Drugs and vaccines

Regarding the therapeutic aspect of the COVID-19 crisis, AI has been employed in three areas: *drug repurposing*, new drug discovery, and vaccine development (Kaushal et al., 2020). Of these three areas, *drug repurposing*, which is the identification of new uses for existing drugs, represents the most researched area (Kaushal et al., 2020).

AI-based *drug repurposing* research generates learning and prediction models that perform *quick screening* of drugs for new applications (Ke et al., 2020). AI-based *drug repurposing* is inexpensive, faster and more efficient than traditional methods (Mohanty et al., 2020). The drugs under study go directly to more advanced stages of testing, as initial tests, such as toxicity tests, are not necessary since it is known how they affect humans

(Kaushal et al., 2020). This process is highly relevant in the context of COVID-19, which is characterized by the need to find solutions as quickly as possible.

The studies by Delijewski and Haneczok (2021) and Ke et al. (2020) are examples of AI-based analyses of the utility against COVID-19 of drugs that are currently marketed to treat other diseases, demonstrating that the application of AI for *drug repurposing* in the framework of COVID-19 is feasible. However, it should be noted that despite the great potential and encouraging results of AI-based *drug repurposing* in the fight against novel coronavirus, this technology is still underdeveloped (Mohanty et al., 2020; Zhou et al., 2020). The low relevance of AI-based *drug repurposing* may be due, as in other AI applications, to the paucity of data (Dotolo et al., 2021).

Regarding research on new drugs against COVID-19, thousands of new potentially effective compounds have been identified by AI at a high rate. However, their clinical efficacy for the treatment of COVID-19 is unknown, and therefore, more research is needed to draw conclusions (Kaushal et al., 2020). Moreover, AI-based applications can reduce the time and cost of drug development (Kaushik and Raj, 2020; Lavecchia, 2019). However, AI has not had a major impact in this area in the context of COVID-19, which again may be due to the paucity of data in this regard (Kaushik and Raj, 2020). What is certain is that *open data sharing* is a key factor for global progress in AI-based pharmacological research (Jiménez-Luna et al., 2021).

The third therapeutic aspect of the COVID-19 crisis to which AI can be applied is vaccine development (Kaushal et al., 2020). AI has been helpful in learning more about the new coronavirus and detecting which components will elicit an immune response, decreasing the time spent in this phase of research (Waltz, 2020). However, AI cannot do anything in clinical trials of the vaccine, where it is necessary to inoculate and test individuals on a voluntary basis (Waltz, 2020).

In the area of COVID-19 vaccines, AI can also be useful for optimizing vaccine distribution. Kumar and Veer (2021) argue that AI could be used to make predictions about the demand for vaccines and, consequently, facilitate decisions about the destination and volume of shipments. It could also help to determine which population groups should be vaccinated first and to monitor the possible occurrence of adverse side effects that have not been identified in clinical trials. This process would support the management of the COVID-19 vaccine supply chain through AI.

Facebook (2021) also proposes using AI-based population density maps to optimize vaccination in sparsely populated areas of the world. They propose that population density maps developed by Facebook have been used successfully before. For example, the American Red Cross and the Malawi Ministry of Health used them during a measles vaccination campaign. Thanks to the maps, they discovered that 97 % of Malawi's land area was uninhabited, and because the vaccination strategy was based on house-to-house visits, the route was optimized and the time needed to vaccinate the population was significantly reduced (Facebook, 2021).

Regarding the analysis of potential vaccine side effects, the method used in most studies is statistical analysis (e.g., Almufty et al., 2021; Klugar et al., 2021; Saeed, 2021). However, AI can also be used to predict the severity of such effects, as Hatmal et al. (2021) have done. Moreover, in November 2020, before the coronavirus vaccination campaign began, the UK *Medicines and Healthcare Products Regulatory Agency* (MHRA) signed a contract with the AI-based solution developer Genpact to create an AI-based COVID-19 vaccine side-effect surveillance system (Kahn, 2020). However, the MHRA has not made a clear statement on the results of this monitoring system (GOV. UK, 2021).

In any case, to investigate possible treatments or applications of AI in the context of COVID-19, it is essential to turn to the specialized literature to discover the studies that have already been conducted and the conclusions that have been drawn from them. This task can be complicated, given the large volume of publications that exist on the subject. AI can be used to facilitate this effort. In particular, *AI-based search tools*, such as WellAI use AI to perform more accurate and efficient searches (Kricka et al., 2020). *AI-based search tools* offer several advantages over conventional scientific publication search engines. Their main goal is to summarize and predict relationships. *AI-based search tools* recognize synonyms and related terms, providing more accurate results than traditional search engines that only display publications containing the keywords entered (Kricka et al., 2020).

Ultimately, during the pandemic, numerous AI-based solutions have been developed to combat COVID-19 at the health care level. The main areas of application are (i) prediction and surveillance of the spread of the coronavirus, (ii) *patient management*, (iii) diagnosis and prognosis of the disease, and (iv) drug and vaccine research. Finally, it should be noted that there are barriers to the application of AI in the health sector. For example, there are limitations regarding the availability and reliability of the data used to train the algorithms (Coombs, 2020). There is also reluctance on the various actors surrounding health care services: health care organizations, health care professionals, providers of AI-based health care applications, and patients (Kannan et al., 2020; Shareef et al., 2021; Xing et al., 2021). Likewise, the ethics associated with AI is an issue that has been and continues to be of current interest both in general and in the context of COVID-19 and may hinder the development of applications to combat the pandemic (Ryan and Stahl, 2021; Sachar et al., 2020).

3.2.2. Education

In 2020, the *International Journal of Educational Technology in Higher Education*, a journal that is positioned in the first quartile (Q1) in the most prestigious international rankings of scientific research journals, called for submissions addressing the use of AI in higher education for a special issue of the journal given the potential that some scholars attribute to this technology to revolutionize the sector. Specifically, the purpose of this special issue was *"to examine the potential and actual impact of artificial intelligence (AI) on teaching and learning in higher education"* (Bates et al., 2020, p. 1). The *International Journal of Educational Technology in Higher Education* received 23 contributions, only four of which were considered to be of appropriate quality for publication (Bates et al., 2020).

This anecdote is indicative of the state of AI in the education sector: despite the potential attributed to AI in this context (Zhang and Aslan, 2021), its adoption in teaching and learning is still at an early stage (Luan et al., 2020). Although there are studies showing the usefulness of AI in education, there is hardly any use of this technology in real educational settings (Kabudi et al., 2021), and its development mainly comes from private companies that, unlike universities, have access to large datasets that make it possible to create scalable and cost-effective AI-based educational systems (Bates et al., 2020). However, it should be noted that research about the use of AI in education has increased since 2018, mainly in the area of *computer science* (Bozkurt et al., 2021).

3.2.2.1. Areas of application

Among the four contributions selected for publication is the systematic review of the use of IL in higher education by Zawacki-Richter et al. (2020). These authors identify four main areas of application of IL in this context: *profiling and prediction, intelligent tutoring systems, assessment and evaluation*, and *adaptive systems and personalization*.

Profiling and prediction refer to the creation of models or profiles of students to predict their risk of dropping out, their likelihood of being admitted and their future performance, among others (Zawacki-Richter et al., 2020). In this area, AI has been used to predict different variables during the pandemic, such as the intention to use *mobile learning platforms* (Akour et al., 2021), students' performance in the COVID-19 context (Tarik et al., 2021) and university students' satisfaction with distance education as a consequence of the coronavirus (Ho et al., 2021).

The data used to make these predictions can come from a variety of sources. For example, before the pandemic, Smirnov (2020) studied the ability to predict through AI the scores of Russian students in the Unified States Examination (USE) (a compulsory exam that students must pass in Russia to enter university) and in the Programme for International Student Assessment (PISA). To do this, it uses data from social media, in particular from student posts on VK (a Russian social network) and Twitter. Aggarwal et al. (2021) combine academic and nonacademic data, such as demographics.

Intelligent tutoring systems are based on AI to decide the *learning path* of each student and select what content is offered progressively. The aim is to help and involve the student in an individualized way, especially in distance courses where many students participate, and it is difficult to offer *one-to-one* human tutoring (Zawacki-Richter et al., 2020). In the context of the pandemic, Mirchi et al. (2020) propose combining *intelligent tutoring systems* with virtual reality simulators for surgical students to continue practicing and developing their skills. These authors claim that pairing *intelligent tutoring systems* with virtual reality simulators provides students with hyperrealistic experiences that, thanks to AI, provide feedback on their performance in surgical practice. This finding could counteract the negative effects that COVID-19 has had on the development of their training.

During this period, Cao et al. (2021) analyze the determinants that explain the adoption of *intelligent tutoring systems* by *college students* in China. After the pandemic began, Chinese authorities implemented a digital education strategy that included the use of *intelligent tutoring systems to ensure* the effectiveness of online tutoring (Cao et al., 2021). From their study, they find that perceived ease of use, perceived usefulness, and students' attitudes, among others, significantly affect students' intention to use these AI-based systems.

Assessment and evaluation refer to the application of AI to automate grading, provide feedback, and evaluate understanding and teaching, among others (Zawacki-Richter et al., 2020). Cope et al. (2020) argue that assessment may be the area that harbors the most opportunities for transforming education through AI. Jena (2020) discusses the effects of COVID-19 on higher education in India and examines its impact, *emerging approaches* during the pandemic and post COVID-19 trends. Among the new trends that he suggests will transform the teaching-learning process is AI-based *assessment and evaluation. In* particular, Jena (2020) contends that AI-based assessment of learners will help reduce the burden on teachers so that they can devote their efforts to other tasks such as course and skill development.

The strategy of social distancing and confinement has forced educational institutions to transfer teaching to the digital plane. This transfer has taken place not only in terms of the delivery of knowledge but also in terms of its assessment. In the period marked by COVID-19, examinations have taken place remotely through digital platforms (Awad Ahmed et al., 2021; Chirumamilla and Sindre, 2021). Some companies have offered their services for free. For example, Gradescope is an online grading tool that uses AI to recognize and grade handwritten text in English and mathematical notation (Gradescope, n.d.). Gradescope is a paid platform but offers services free of charge to teachers from March until December 2020 to help them adapt to distance teaching and assessment (Gradescope, 2020).

Most of the teachers were inexperienced in this regard, and there was a possibility that students might engage in irregular practices to obtain better grades on the exam (Bilen and Matros, 2021). Therefore, some educational institutions resorted to various e-monitoring technologies to track online examinations and ensure academic integrity (Kharbat and Daabes, 2021). Some e-supervision systems are AI-based, such as the SwiftAssess AI Proctor, which is a feature of SwiftAsses, a cloud-based assessment management platform that monitors online assessments through AI. This system *can be implemented in any public, private cloud or dedicated server*. It is able to detect suspicious actions such as *absent students, unauthorized persons, incorrect gaze, window changing and screen sharing*. To do this, AI Proctor verifies the identity of the student taking the test and takes information through the microphone and camera of the device from which the test is taken. The teacher decides whether he or she prefers the system to send real-time alerts when a suspicious event is discovered or to receive a report at the end of the exam (GamaLearn, 2021).

Finally, the area of *adaptive systems and personalization* encompasses teaching content and its recommendation, as well as the use of academic data to monitor and guide students and design courses (Zawacki-Richter et al., 2020). Through IL, it would be possible to personalize training provision and tailor it to learners' prior knowledge and experience. AI could make it possible to recognize knowledge gaps and detect what content to provide for each learner (Schlegelmilch, 2020). Knewton and Connect are two examples of AI-based platforms that improve student performance through *personalized learning* (Kabudi et al., 2021).

Notably, these four areas may be complementary and that several of them may be present in the same AI-based educational application. Education is evolving from a *one-size-fits-all* approach to a more personalized model that considers the individual differences of each learner (Luan et al., 2020). AI can help to identify the profile of each student to provide *intelligent tutoring* and *adaptive teaching*, automate assessments and provide *feedback* to each student through AI.

3.2.2.2. Barriers and digital transformation process

There are, however, barriers that hinder the expansion of IL in higher education. Elhajjar et al. (2021) name the following: the shortage of funds to provide the necessary technological infrastructure, the lack of skills and competencies among faculty, and resistance to change. Moreover, Elhajjar et al. (2021) detect that members of the university community consider that higher education institutions are not ready to adopt IL within academic courses and that a possible solution lies in collaboration with companies in the technology sector. In this sense, Asakura et al. (2020) narrate how they partnered with a company in the technology sector to develop a virtual platform based on AI for their students to practice their skills.

The truth is that AI-based educational applications such as those mentioned above are usually from private companies and are paid for (e.g., Gradescope and Knewton). Developing AI-based applications is a complex process. However, there are resources available that can simplify it. For example, the technology company that partnered with Asakura et al. (2020) for the creation of an AI-based educational platform made use of IBM Watson Assistant, one of the products offered by IBM Watson, an AI-based system developed by IBM. IBM Watson is defined as "*IBM's portfolio of business-ready tools, applications and solutions, designed to reduce the costs and hurdles of AI adoption while optimizing outcomes and responsible use of AI*" (IBM, n.d.). Its clients include KPMG and Thomson Reuters (IBM, n.d.).

The pandemic has also accelerated the process of digital transformation in the education sector. Educational leaders and teachers have been forced to continue the academic year digitally as a result of confinement and social distancing measures to curb the spread of the virus. This new means of teaching presents an opportunity to digitize education and embrace the resources available in the 21st century.

Krishnamurthy (2020) proposes that the transition to online learning as a result of COVID-19 should be divided into three phases: *instructional continuity, instructional design* and *AI-enabled innovation*. The first phase, *instructional continuity*, refers to the need to ensure that students have access to learning during the coronavirus crisis and to adopt mechanisms in the short term that allow courses to be offered remotely. The second phase, *instructional design*, focuses on improving the learning experience by introducing digital tools that reinforce the new *online* learning system. Finally, in the third phase, *AI-enabled innovation*, Krishnamurthy (2020) advocates the use of AI-based services within the teaching process as the new normal after the coronavirus crisis. These AI-based innovations are aimed at transforming the educational experience as we know it today.

In conclusion, IL has great potential to improve the teaching-learning process. The implementation of IL in education and research is still in its infancy (Luan et al., 2020). However, the pandemic has accelerated the digital transformation of this sector. Educational leaders have turned to a variety of digital tools, some of them AI-based, to continue education during the period of uncertainty caused by COVID-19. Some paid AI-based education apps, such as Gradescope, have offered free access to their services to help mitigate the negative effects of the new coronavirus on education.

3.2.3. Other

COVID-19 has meant a paradigm shift for companies and the way they operate. According to a study by Anderson et al. (2021), the pandemic has accelerated the digital transformation of 59 % of companies. Companies, in addition to developing AI-based applications to help in the fight against COVID-19, such as body temperature detectors and facial recognition (Kang et al., 2021), have also introduced AI into their own processes during this period.

AI has improved the competitiveness of some companies in the context of COVID-19. In particular, according to a study by Xu et al. (2021), the revenues of companies that used AI before the pandemic increased faster in 2020 than those that did not. Given the potential for AI to create opportunities during the pandemic, Sipior (2020) advocates the creation of a *Chief AI Officer* (CIAO). Unlike the Chief Information Officer (CIO), who focuses on the delivery of *IT services* and their impact on business performance, the CIAO would be responsible for identifying where AI could be introduced, overseeing its implementation and monitoring its performance.

AI represents an opportunity to improve different processes carried out by companies. For example, AI can help build the resilience of supply chains in the context of uncertainty caused by COVID-19 (Modgil et al., 2021). Similarly, several hotels in China have used AI to improve service quality during the pandemic. In particular, they have used facial recognition technology to improve the efficiency and ease of customer *check-in* and *check-out* processes (Lau, 2020).

AI can also be used to improve customer service. Telefónica, a Spanish telecommunications company that operates internationally, has used AI to improve its customer service and prioritize customers over the age of 65 during the pandemic. Telefónica argues that older people are more at risk of being victims of phone fraud in the context of the pandemic. Therefore, they turned to Nuance, a company that develops AI-based solutions, to implement a system that identifies an individual's age through voice recognition. Thanks to this system, they were able to prioritize calls from people over 65 and improve the quality of the service provided (Nuance, 2020).

The new coronavirus has changed consumer habits and accelerated the growth of e-commerce (Guthrie et al., 2021). In this area, AI can be applied to the development of recommendation systems adapted to the characteristics of each buyer. This finding can help to increase sales, increase the accuracy of sales predictions and reduce the cost of inventory (Zhang and Lu, 2021).

AI also has the potential to be applied to analyze the relationships between variables related to employee performance and to make predictions of future employee behavior. The main obstacle for companies to develop this type of study through AI was the scarcity of data, since before the pandemic, much information was not usually recorded. The implementation of teleworking as a consequence of the pandemic and confinement has created an opportunity to access and store this information. These *datasets* that include different variables that quantify the actions of workers can be used to feed AI algorithms and make predictions about how employees will behave in different situations, which would facilitate organizational decision-making and business management (Leonardi, 2021).

3.2.3.1. Social media and misinformation

As in previous epidemics such as Ebola, yellow fever and Zika, the spread of COVID-19 has been accompanied by the spread of *misinformation* (Shahi et al., 2021). *Misinformation* is false or misleading information, regardless of whether there are ill intentions in spreading it (Southwell et al., 2019). The main channel through which *misinformation* about COVID-19 has been spread is *social media*. *Sylvie Briand, director of Infectious Hazards Management at WHO's Health Emergencies Programme*, states: *"with social media is that this phenomenon [misinformation] is amplified, it goes faster and further, like the viruses that travel with people and go faster and further"* (Zarocostas, 2020, p. 676).

Misinformation in health emergencies, such as that caused by COVID-19, can lead people to behave in ways that threaten their own health and the healths of others. For example, some home remedies, such as vitamin C or garlic, have been reported to prevent COVID-19 infection, although there is no scientific evidence to support these claims (Mian and Khan, 2020). Following these false recommendations from social networks can cause a feeling of invulnerability, as the person who follows the recommendation thinks that he or she will not contract the disease and consequently acts recklessly by exposing himself or herself to the virus and could infect third parties. Other supposed remedies against COVID-19 can cause serious damage. This case is true for *chlorine dioxide*, whose popularity grew rapidly on social networks. This compound can cause vomiting, life-threatening hypotension and acute liver failure. The risk is such that the *American Food and Drug Administration* has issued several warnings about it to raise public awareness (Mian and Khan, 2020).

Misinformation can also lead to mistrust of those responsible for pandemic management and negatively affect the efforts of health professionals (Guarino et al., 2021). These consequences make health *misinformation a* public health problem (Zhou et al., 2021a). Such *misinformation* about COVID-19 has led to the coining of the term *infodemic, which refers* to this phenomenon (Zarocostas, 2020). In this context, creating strategies to curb the spread of *misinformation* is of great importance, for which AI can be used. Choudrie et al. (2021) analyze the ability of AI to distinguish between truthful information and fake news about COVID-19 prevention and cure. In their study, they found that AI is able to differentiate between the two with high accuracy (over 85 %). AI is also able to predict whether users will share information from unreliable sources (Mu and Aletras, 2020), helping to identify which profiles are more likely to engage in this practice.

Some of the most important social networks have used this technology to fight *misinformation*. For example, Facebook, one of the most important social networks, has been fighting against *misinformation* since before the COVID-19 pandemic. More than 60 companies work for Facebook to check the veracity of the information shared on this platform. When an image is labeled as *misinformation*, Facebook does not delete it but displays a label to warn its users. In the context of COVID-19 and *infodemics*, the analysis of such a volume of information requires a greater number of resources.

Therefore, Facebook has turned to AI to *scale* the work of its external reviewers. Specifically, it has used existing AI applications and developed new ones to detect copies of posts that its external reviewers have flagged as *misinformation* and stop them from spreading. These AI systems compare images and look for similarities between them to identify copies of those previously flagged as fake by reviewers. Thanks to this technology, Facebook warned of the falsity of 50 million instances of COVID-19–related content in April 2020 based on 7,500 articles checked by reviewers (Facebook, 2020).

Twitter, another popular social network, increased its use of AI in March 2020 to identify potentially manipulative content. However, Twitter is aware that AI can make classification errors due to a lack of context sometimes being present. Therefore, content that has been flagged as suspicious is subjected to human review before Twitter permanently suspends an account (Twitter, 2020).

The truth is that a large percentage of the population uses social media, both to share news and information and to express their own opinions and thoughts. In the context of the pandemic, analyzing the comments posted on social networks about the situation regarding the new coronavirus can be very helpful. Knowing what the public thinks about the pandemic and its management can facilitate the development of more effective public policies and communication campaigns (Flint et al., 2021; Hung et al., 2020), which can also be accomplished through AI. Proof of this concept is shown in the study by Hung et al. (2020), who used AI to analyze the comments posted on Twitter at the beginning of the pandemic. Specifically, they study the subject matter and sentiments (positive, neutral or negative) of the *tweets*. Moreover, Madani et al. (2021) employ AI to detect fake news on Twitter during the COVID-19 period and conclude that *the sentiment of tweets plays an important role in the detection of fake news.*

Thus, COVID-19 has been an unprecedented crisis that has forced the scientific community to work at great speed to learn more about the new virus and to implement measures to curb its spread. In this context, *mis-information* has put at risk the health of citizens who have had difficulty detecting what information was truthful. Thanks to AI, it has been possible to combat the spread of *misinformation* and prevent the population from engaging in behaviors that could negatively affect their health.

4. Gamification and artificial intelligence applications during the COVID-19 crisis

4.1. Introduction

The previous chapters have dealt with the use of gamification and AI during the pandemic. Next, we will analyze the union of both in the health and educational fields during the same period. While there are proposals in the literature that bring together gamification and AI from a practical point of view (e.g., Konstantakopoulos et al., 2019; Polito and Temperini, 2021; Tan and Cheah, 2021), the systematic study of their convergence is practically nonexistent. To our knowledge, the work of Khakpour and Colomo-Palacios (2021) is the first published systematic review concerning the convergence of gamification and *machine learning* (ML), which is a *subset* of AI.

Khakpour and Colomo-Palacios (2021) analyze the areas of application of ML in gamification and point out three main areas: learning, personalization and behavioral change. Learning represents the most researched area and encompasses the introduction of ML in gamified systems developed in the educational context with the aim of maintaining students' interest over time. Personalization refers to the use of ML to offer a personalized gamified experience to each user and encourage long-term *engagement through* the modification of the activity. The application in behavioral change refers to the use of ML to vary the gamified design so that the user interacts in a certain way with the gamified system and realizes a change in their behavior.

Khakpour and Colomo-Palacios (2021) also examine the use of gamification in ML and conclude that its most important application is to encourage participation to achieve more data that, in turn, feed the algorithm and improve its performance. With this same purpose, Chen et al. (2020) propose an innovative way of encouraging participation to achieve a greater volume of data to feed the algorithm: developing a multiplayer game. Although it is not gamification but a game in itself, the proposal of Chen et al. (2020) can serve as inspiration to introduce a gamified design in the interactions between users and an AI system.

In the health care field, gamified applications based on AI have been developed in recent years. For example, Goswami et al. (2019) combined gamification and AI in an app for treating snoring and improving sleep quality. Thanks to the development of AI, there are now apps available to the population in the area of health care, which have been of great help during the pandemic. One of them is Fitbod, a gamified AI-based app dedicated to physical activity. AI offers a personalized training plan for each user. It utilizes an algorithm that, based on the data of each individual such as skills and previous workouts, provides a plan tailored to their capabilities. In addition, it encourages *engagement* and, therefore, its continued use through a gamified design.

The level of physical activity in the population has been affected by COVID-19 and the rise of sedentary lifestyles in the context of confinement. Many gyms closed their doors during the first months of the pandemic to help slow the spread of the virus, affecting the level of physical activity of the population. For this reason, Fitbod decided to offer its services free of charge during the period from March 19 to June 1, 2020, and, in this way, help maintain the health of the population (Fitbod, 2021).

Gamified systems based on AI have also been developed in the educational field. However, it should be noted that, in this context, universities seem to contribute less than private companies. Gamified AI applications used in real teaching environments are usually created by technology companies. The applications from the university context found in the literature are proposals that have been tested on small groups of students. For example, Polito and Temperini (2021) developed a system for automated assessment in a gamified learning environment. Twelve students have registered in the system they have created, but only 10 of them participate through it. Tan and Cheah (2021) created a prototype of a gamified platform based on AI and tested its operation on a group of 24 students.

In contrast, there are AI-based gamified educational platforms created by companies with thousands of users, such as the two discussed later in this chapter: Century and ELSA Speak. While these platforms provide paid services, some, such as Century and Fitbod in the health care sector, have offered their services for free during the pandemic to support society and mitigate the damage caused by the coronavirus.

Below are four projects that integrate gamification and AI and have been used during the pandemic to address the effects caused by COVID-19. Two of them, DreamLab: Corona-AI and uMore, are framed within the health field, and the other two, Century and ELSA Speak, are in the educational field. Some had already been developed before the pandemic, and others were developed during this period in response to the new coronavirus, but all have been relevant at this time of uncertainty.

4.2. Applications in health

4.2.1. DreamLab: Corona-AI

DreamLab is a Vodafone Foundation platform that harnesses the processing power of *smartphones*, even though these devices are not in use to accelerate scientific research. Specifically, DreamLab was created in 2015 in collaboration with the Garvan Institute of Medical Research in Australia to help cancer research (Garvan Institute, 2021). This platform is based on distributed computing, through which a significant volume of *computing power* is obtained using several machines that are interconnected (Ramon-Cortes et al., 2021). In the case of DreamLab, the machines are the smartphones of the users who download the app and participate in it voluntarily.

In April 2020, following the onset of the COVID-19 pandemic, the Corona-AI project was launched. Corona-AI is the result of DreamLab's collaboration with researchers from Imperial College London. The two entities had previously collaborated on the DRUGS (Drug Repositioning Using Grids of Smartphones) project, which is framed around cancer research (Veselkov et al., 2019).

The goal of Corona-AI is to examine the potential effect of molecules present in food and drugs on disease caused by COVID-19. These analyses are carried out by millions of mathematical calculations using AI. Given that this requires a large processing capacity, the collaboration of citizens is requested to create a virtual supercomputer thanks to the processing capacity of their mobile phones (Vodafone, 2020).

4.2.1.1. *DreamLab: Corona-AI during the COVID-19*

The research conducted through Corona-AI was initially postponed due to the limited computing capacity available to them (Veselkov, 2020).

Therefore, they decided to collaborate with the DreamLab platform to access the capacity of thousands of mobile phones. DreamLab is a preexisting platform that was created before the pandemic. That is, the Imperial College London researchers in charge of coronavirus AI research took a previously developed resource and used it to carry out their project focused on COVID-19.

This project has been a success. Thanks to the voluntary participation of the crowd, the first phase of the Corona-AI project was completed in just six months. If the mathematical calculations of this research had been conducted in the traditional way instead of through the DreamLab platform, much more time would have been needed (Vodafone, 2020). This finding is highly relevant in the context of the pandemic, as knowledge about the new coronavirus needs to be advanced very quickly to be able to take effective measures to stop its spread.

By December 2020, eight months after the launch of Corona-AI, almost one million people from 17 countries had downloaded the DreamLab app (Vodafone, 2020). In January 2021, the results of the first phase of the study (see Laponogov et al., 2021) were published. During this period, the second and third phases of the project were completed, and by September 2021, the fourth phase of Corona-AI had almost been completed.

4.2.1.2. Gamification and AI in DreamLab: Corona-AI

Individuals who decide to collaborate with the Corona-AI project should download the DreamLab app on their *smartphones*. It should be noted that this app is free. After that, they must choose which project they want to participate in since DreamLab develops other research in addition to Corona-AI.

In this case, the gamified design is in the DreamLab app. That is, all the projects hosted in it (including Corona-AI) benefit from the effects of gamification on user motivation. The app shows what percentage of each project has been completed, which entity is responsible and its geographical scope. In the case of coronavirus AI, the responsible entity is Imperial College London, and its scope is worldwide. When you select the project you wish to collaborate on, DreamLab presents its mission and statistics. The statistics for each project include the total calculations required for the research, the calculations that have been carried out through DreamLab and the total number of individuals who have collaborated.

The "My Contribution" tab of the app shows the cumulative time during which the user has supported causes through DreamLab and the total number of calculations made. It also displays these statistics broken down by cause. In addition, DreamLab has a design that shows illustrations of scientists, bringing the user closer to the scientific purpose of the app.

In terms of AI, Corona-AI analyses the response of combinations of molecules to SARS-CoV-2, the coronavirus responsible for the pandemic. More technically, Michael Bronstein, a member of the project, explains that Corona-AI employs *"a novel class of network-based AI methods to identify antiviral compounds among a dataset of thousands of molecules, by modeling the network effects of the interactions between these molecules and biomolecules in our body"* (Veselkov, 2020).

The process by which a user wishes to participate in the project is as follows. After downloading the DreamLab app, you must turn it on at night while you are sleeping and your mobile phone is idle and charging. DreamLab only works if the device is connected to the main power source to avoid damaging its battery life. In addition, it needs to have access to the internet, either through a mobile network or Wi-Fi. During these hours, the phone downloads small problems, performs calculations and sends the results to the researchers via the app. In this way, the data processing effort required for the research is divided among thousands of devices, and therefore, the time required to complete the task is greatly reduced (Vodafone, 2021).

The altruistic objective of Corona-AI, together with the gamified design of DreamLab, motivates the participation of users. On the one hand, co-ronavirus AI is researching new ways to treat COVID-19. Helping in this research is free and requires no effort; it simply requires that the DreamLab app be downloaded and activated while the user sleeps. On the other hand, displaying statistics about the time spent collaborating in the project and the number of calculations that have been made thanks to their contribution, as well as the percentage of the project that has been completed, can encourage users to continue collaborating. In addition, illustrations of scientists could help communicate the goals of these projects: scientific research and the advancement of knowledge.

4.2.2. uMore app

uMore is an app dedicated to mental wellbeing created during the pandemic. This app is based on AI and gamification to encourage the adoption of positive habits and, thus, an improvement in the mental health of its users. uMore is able to quantify progress in mental wellbeing. AI offers personalized recommendations to each user based on their state and goals so that they are able to manage their stress and anxiety (uMore, 2020a).

uMore visually displays the user's progress, helping them to understand their progress and motivating them to continue adopting positive habits. To achieve changes in behavior, it uses *cognitive behavioral therapy*, *acceptance and commitment therapy*, *mindfulness*, and *behavioral science* techniques, and through AI, it develops personalized plans for each individual (uMore, 2020b). It is worth noting that uMore is a free app; any individual can download and use it without any cost.

4.2.2.1. *uMore during the COVID*

uMore was created to provide mental health support to COVID-19 patients during their period of isolation. Unlike Corona-AI, which used a preexisting platform, uMore is a project that was created from scratch as a result of COVID-19. According to Maria Freitas, CEO of uMore, the idea arose from the mental health problems of her sister caused by isolation when she became ill with COVID-19 (uMore, 2020c). This occurrence motivated her to participate with a group of friends in a competition organized by the NHS in the United Kingdom that sought proposals to combat the effects of the pandemic, creating the uMore prototype (Gibbon, 2020).

The aim of this app is to destigmatize mental health and provide tools for its users to understand and manage their mental health problems regardless of their location, especially those who suffer from COVID-19 and are isolated (uMore, 2020c).

Thanks to the work of an international team of *product designers, digital technologists,* and *behavioral scientists*, uMore was launched in December 2020 (uMore, 2020c). A few months later, in April 2021, it already had more than 3,000 users, placing it within the *top 50 health and fitness apps in the UAE* (de Freitas, 2021).

uMore has achieved several accomplishments since its inception that attest to its innovative character. For example, it won the 14th Edition of the MIT Enterprise Forum Arab Startup Competition in 2021, an annual competition organized by MIT Enterprise Pan Arab Forum that rewards innovation and entrepreneurship in the *Arab Region* (MIT Enterprise Forum, n.d.). uMore has also received funding from TheVenturCity, a company that invests in innovative startups (TheVentureCity, 2021) and is one of 10 projects selected to participate in "Growth Academy: Health & Wellbeing," a program created by Google that offers mentoring with Google employees and industry experts to facilitate the growth of startups (Benjumea, 2021).

4.2.2.2. Gamification and AI in uMore

uMore conducts daily tracking and sends notifications to users to remind them of what habits they want to improve and when to take an assessment of their state of mental wellbeing. uMore claims that through this continuous monitoring, a sense of achievement and *cognitive closure* is generated (uMore, 2020d).

Specifically, this application is based on the *habit loop* to reinforce this change in behavior. The *habit loop* is a mechanism by which an action is rewarded after carrying it out. In the case of uMore, the trigger of this *loop* is the notification sent by the app. After that, the user carries out the activities recommended through AI by the app and the evaluation of his state of mental well-being. The reward they receive in return is their score and the visualization of their progress over time. This reward encourages continued use of the app and the acquisition of positive habits. In addition, the results can be shared with loved ones or even a doctor if their app accounts are linked (uMore, 2020d).

Maria de Freitas, CEO of uMore, defines this app as the *"Fitbit for feelings"* (Gibbon, 2020). Fitbit is a technology company dedicated to health and physical activity. It is one of the most popular *wearable companies* that measure physical activity using smart watches and bracelets (Fitbit, 2021). To encourage user engagement and incentivize their continued use in the long term, Fitbit's app has a gamified design that has been widely analyzed in the specialized literature (e.g., Bitrián et al., 2021; Chung et al., 2017; Huang et al., 2019).

uMore, like Fitbit, makes use of gamification. The uMore app provides users with information about their current state of mental health and their progress over time in a visual way. Stress, anxiety and depression levels are displayed through bar graphs. The overall wellbeing score, which can be understood as points in a gamified design, is displayed in a pie chart. Progress in the level of stress, well-being and mood is also presented. The latter is measured through *emojis* that represent the user's feelings.

Although uMore does not explicitly state it, this gamified design is what the app's website calls a reward. In the *habit loop* on which the app is based, these rewards encourage continued use and, as a result, the acquisition of positive habits (uMore, 2020d). In other words, in this case, gamification is used as a technique to encourage participation in this AI-based app and as an incentive for users to adopt habits that positively affect their mental health.

Through AI, uMore creates personalized plans for each user based on their state. To do this, the app employs techniques from *cognitive behavioral therapy, acceptance and commitment therapy, mindfulness,* and *behavioral science* (uMore, 2020b). uMore not only measures the level of stress, as do other mental health apps, but also asks questions about the user's mood to improve its understanding of each individual's situation and provide recommendations that fit their particular circumstances (Gibbon, 2020).

4.3. Applications in education

4.3.1. Century

Century is a gamified educational platform created in 2013 that combines learning science, AI and neuroscience. Century aims to help both teachers and students. Through AI, it provides personalized learning based on the knowledge, skills, learning pace and *learning gaps* of each student. Through this technology, real-time statistics about student performance and behavior is provided to teachers, helping to reduce their workload (Century, 2021a).

Century is a paid platform and is aimed at all educational levels, as well as training within the business world. It is present in 45 countries around the world (Century, 2021b) and is used in a multitude of educational institutions, among them Eton College, an important school in the

UK where *20 prime ministers* have studied (Century, 2021c), which has been using Century since 2019.

4.3.1.1. *Century during COVID-19*

Century was created in 2013, long before the pandemic. Therefore, unlike the previous example in health care, it is a preexisting platform. However, it has been a great help for many schools in different countries to continue with their online teaching process during the period marked by COVID-19. Proof of this is that the use of Century increased by 400 % in 2020 (UKTN, 2021).

Century is a paid platform but has offered its services for free during the pandemic to help teachers and students around the world. The first people Century wanted to help were teachers and students at schools in China, where the epicenter of the pandemic was located. It then extended the offer to Hong Kong. By February 12, 2020, 25 schools had applied for free access to the platform (Hazell, 2020). Gradually, the list of schools and countries incorporating Century into their strategy for adapting to online learning during the pandemic expanded. China and Hong Kong were joined by Vietnam, South Korea, Japan, Thailand and the UAE. By March 5, 2020, 50 schools were using Century free of charge (Anderson, 2020). The offer was then extended to Italy and the rest of Europe (Epstein, 2020). In May 2020, the *Lebanese Ministry of Education and Higher Education* and the *UK government's Department for International Development* agreed to provide Century services free of charge to public schools in Lebanon (Century, 2020).

Priya Lakhani, CEO of Century, argues that on the one hand, they have lost tens of thousands of euros by offering free access to the platform. On the other hand, in addition to helping many schools, teachers and students during this period of uncertainty, this decision also had a positive effect on the company. Thanks to this, a large number of potential customers have become aware of their services. In addition, they have moved up the adoption curve, moving beyond the early adopter phase. Their offering has been so well received that they have had to double their servers to cope with the demand, which has increased by 400 % during 2020 (Epstein, 2020; UKTN, 2021).

Century has continued to grow through 2021, receiving $6.5 million in funding (UKTN, 2021). Part of this investment comes from the Solve Innovation Future, a *philanthropic venture fund* that is part of a Massachusetts Institute of Technology (MIT) initiative whose mission is to solve grand global challenges through social impact innovation (Snyder, 2021). The Solve Innovation Future *raises funds from philanthropic donors and MIT*, which acts as an advisor to donors, that are invested in the selected Solver teams (MIT Solve, 2021).

4.3.1.2. *Gamification and AI in century*

Century aims to solve two problems: student boredom and excessive teacher workload (Anderson, 2020). Thanks to AI, this platform enables personalized learning and reduces the burden on teachers. Moreover, possessing a gamified design motivates students and generates their interest. Century uses a dashboard to show each student's progress using a score, the percentage of skills they have acquired, their grade in the diagnostic tasks and the percentage of the task they have completed, among others, which encourages them to continue interacting within the platform and improve their performance.

Regarding AI, Century introduces it within it to differentiate itself from other educational apps. At its inception, its founder wondered how she could convince schools and teachers to use her platform. According to her, there are many digital education apps out there, and many of them work very well. Therefore, she thought Century should incorporate AI to offer something more than the competition. His idea was to create a platform that would provide real-time data about student behavior that would allow them to improve the teaching-learning process (Lynley, 2016).

Century works as follows. First, teachers can select a lesson from those available on the platform or upload their own content. Then, students begin to engage with the material, and by analyzing their actions and performance, Century learns the level of knowledge, skills, learning pace and *gaps* of each. Based on these parameters, the platform offers a personalized learning path and helps to understand the content in which each student needs to dedicate more effort. In addition, it provides real-time information to teachers so that they can know at any time the performance level of their students and can help them in their learning process (Anderson, 2020; Century, 2021a). Thanks to this monitoring and notification system for teachers, the company claims that it can reduce the workload of teachers by up to 6 hours per week (Century, 2021c).

Gamification and AI are combined within this platform to create an interesting and motivating experience that fosters student *engagement* and enhances their learning process through personalization. This personalization is very important in the context of COVID-19, when teaching moved to the digital plane and caused challenges for school leaders, teachers and students alike. However, the implementation of Century may cause concern and reluctance among school leaders and teachers, who may be unfamiliar with how such platforms work and fear their potential complexity. This issue can be exacerbated during the pandemic because, while these resources can be helpful, their implementation takes place while schools are closed and education takes place at a distance. As such, platforms need to simplify this process. In the case of Century, implementation can be completed in three hours. In addition, they advise assigning a project manager to act as a link between Century and the families and, in this way, facilitate communication between the parties (Lieberman, 2020).

4.3.2. ELSA Speak

ELSA Speak (an acronym for English Learning Speech Assistant) is an app that helps improve English pronunciation for individuals who are not native speakers of English. ELSA Speak is based on AI. This app uses speech recognition to detect the mistakes made by the user and provide the appropriate corrections (ELSA Speak, n.d.).

ELSA Speak was created in 2016, and two years later, in 2018, it had millions of users from 100 countries (Gilchrist, 2020). The app is free to download. However, a fee must be paid to access the services within it. This fee can be an annual or quarterly subscription. It is currently available in nine languages (*English, Hindi, Indonesian, Japanese, Korea, Portuguese, Spanish, Thai* and *Vietnamese*) and plans to continue to add more languages (ELSA Speak, 2020c).

4.3.2.1. ELSA Speak during COVID-19

As mentioned above, ELSA Speak is a platform that was created in 2016, several years before the COVID-19 outbreak. It is a preexisting platform that, moreover, has not been modified to be used during the period marked by the new coronavirus since it has maintained the same functionalities that it already offered previously.

The pandemic, and more specifically confinement, has meant a change in teaching processes, which have had to adapt to online teaching and use digital tools. In the case of ELSA Speak, the number of users has multiplied three to four times each month during the pandemic (Gilchrist, 2020). In addition, the app has accessed new types of users during the pandemic. Before the pandemic, ELSA Speak targeted individuals who wanted to improve their English pronunciation. With the closure of schools, educational institutions in different countries, such as Vietnam, India and Brazil, have partnered with them to continue teaching English to their students through this app (Gilchrist, 2020).

Furthermore, in March 2020, following the outbreak of the pandemic, ELSA Speak offered the use of the app free of charge to students at all levels of education anywhere in the world until June 30, 2020. This offer was intended to curb the adverse effects that COVID-19 had on student learning (ELSA Speak, 2020a, b).

4.3.2.2. Gamification and AI in ELSA Speak

According to Vu Van, cofounder of ELSA Speak, what determines the success of an app is its ability to keep users interested (Tran, 2019). There is little point in attracting new users and increasing the volume of downloads of the app if they do not continue to use it. In this sense, gamification can be of great help, as it aims to motivate individuals and encourage behavioral change. The ELSA Speak app has a gamified design that shows users' progress through scores and percentages. In addition, it develops a narrative through images and illustrations.

In terms of AI, this platform bases its operation on voice recognition, through which ELSA Speak is able to detect and correct the pronunciation errors of its users. When the ELSA Speak prototype was created, the company's founders had to train the algorithm on which the app is based through data. The founders struggled to input data from nonnative English speakers and compare it to U.S. English. To do this, they turned to individuals from Vietnam, the home country of one of the founders. It was essential to collect data quickly; the speed with which the algorithm is trained depends on how quickly data is collected and, therefore, the time needed to optimize the functioning of the app (Gilchrist, 2020).

A few months later, ELSA Speak won a *startup* competition. This win resulted in 30,000 new users in 24 hours, which was a great opportunity to obtain more data and improve the AI on which ELSA Speak is based (Gilchrist, 2020). This improvement continues to take place today. The capability of the AI on which ELSA Speak is based improves if the number of users increases and they come from different countries as the algorithm is still being trained. In addition, these users must actively use the app to obtain the data to feed the algorithm. In this scenario, gamification plays an important role in encouraging the use of ELSA Speak and facilitating its continued improvement.

5. Ethical issues in gamification and artificial intelligence during the COVID-19 crisis

5.1. Introduction

The pandemic has raised difficult ethical decisions, mainly in the health care domain, such as fairness in the distribution of scarce medical supplies and in deciding whom to prioritize in providing treatment, which lead health care professionals into tough moral conflicts (Arora and Arora, 2020; Kim and Grady, 2020; Turale et al., 2020). Likewise, ethics management has also been present in the applications on which this book focuses: the applications integrating gamification and AI employed during the COVID-19 crisis.

As discussed throughout this book, gamification and AI have been of great importance in the development of solutions to combat the effects of the new coronavirus. One of the main means through which they have been employed has been digital applications and platforms. The first ethical problem that arises in these circumstances is a consequence of the digital divide. The digital divide refers to the disparity of the capabilities and resources to access and employ digital technology (Gran et al., 2021). Although gamification and AI can help mitigate the effects of the pandemic, these innovations are of little use if a sector of the population cannot access them. Moreover, from an ethical point of view, the inability to enjoy these services may harm the most vulnerable population. These disparities may have been aggravated during COVID-19.

Moreover, the study of the ethics surrounding AI is a topic that has been of interest since before and during the pandemic (Ryan and Stahl, 2021; Sachar et al., 2020). AI-based systems developed to combat COVID-19 must follow ethical principles and respect human rights (Luego-Oroz et al., 2020). However, the need to find solutions in a short time to address COVID-19 may cause the ethical application of AI to be neglected. Tzachor et al. (2020) warn of this risk and highlight the importance of analyzing the ethical aspects of AI implementation in the context of the pandemic as a matter of urgency. To this end, they encourage technologists, ethicists, policy-makers and health care professionals to participate in this work and to become involved in the development of analyses that avoid neglecting the ethics surrounding AI during the crisis triggered by COVID-19.

Moreover, many AI applications have been developed in the health care sector. Quinn et al. (2021) highlight three major challenges facing AI in its application in this field: conceptual challenges, technical challenges, and humanistic challenges. Conceptual challenges refer to the complexity involved in the approach to the problem to be solved by AI. Technical challenges refer to the difficulty of practically implementing AI-based health care applications. Finally, humanistic challenges are those related to the social and ethical implications of the use of AI in health care services. In this regard, the lack of transparency in the operation of algorithms, enhanced by their high complexity, has important ethical implications and represents an obstacle to their use in real settings (Linardatos et al., 2021; Walmsley, 2021).

As discussed in the previous chapter, some AI-based systems include a gamified design that encourages participation. The purpose in these cases may be to obtain more data to be able to analyze them and make predictions using AI. In this context, ethical dilemmas regarding whether individual privacy or the common good should be prioritized, such as in public health, arise (Latif et al., 2020). In the face of the health emergency caused by COVID-19, the question regarding whether data, even sensitive data, such as clinical data, should be shared to expedite the development of solutions arises. In addition, while gamification encourages participation in these applications, it may also jeopardize the protection of individual privacy.

Given the above, this chapter focuses on the ethical challenges posed by the use of gamification and AI in the context of the COVID-19 pandemic. Specifically, this chapter addresses the ethical implications of the digital divide, the transparency of these applications, the protection of individuals' privacy, and the legal framework in which they are developed.

5.2. Digital divide

As has been presented through different arguments and examples throughout this book, gamification and AI supported by digital technology have been applied during the COVID-19 crisis. For gamification and AI to be useful during this period, it is key that the users of these applications possess electronic devices with internet access and have the necessary capabilities to use them. However, not all the population has these resources and capabilities. This is the so-called digital divide.

Gran et al. (2021) identify three levels within the digital divide. The first level refers to the ability of access to infrastructure. Infrastructure encompasses both digital devices (such as computers, smartphones and tablets) and internet connections. The second level of the digital divide refers to the skills and capabilities needed to use digital technology. Finally, the third level addresses whether these skills and abilities are beneficial (Gran et al., 2021). It should be noted that some sectors of the population are more affected by the digital divide, which has been aggravated during COVID-19. These include residents of rural areas (Lai and Widmar, 2021), elderly individuals (Van Jaarsveld, 2020) and inhabitants of low- and middle-income countries (Kumm et al., 2021).

Given the above, the digital divide represents an obstacle for the population to take advantage of the AI-based gamified solutions created in the framework of the pandemic, both in the health care and educational domains. Ethical problems emerge when individuals cannot access these applications and no solution is offered. This is compounded when essential services such as health care and education are provided through them. While gamification and AI possess great potential to help mitigate the effects of COVID-19, they can also worsen the disparities between different population groups and widen the gap experienced by the most vulnerable population groups.

With regard to health care, the lack of electronic devices and internet connectivity does not allow the full potential of digital health initiatives aimed at continuing remote health care during the pandemic to be realized (Clare, 2021). As a result, the digital divide during COVID-19 has exacerbated existing disparities between the most vulnerable sectors and the rest of the population in terms of access to and quality of health care (Eruchalu et al., 2021). One possible solution in this regard is to offer health care via telephone. However, it should be noted that this is a short-term solution to soften the effects of COVID-19 mitigation measures since telephone consultations limit interactions between doctors and patients who can only communicate in spoken form (Saeed and Masters, 2021).

Beyond the limitation of access to technology and the lack of skills to employ it, there is another barrier associated with digital applications: lack of trust. AI-based health care applications face the challenge of generating trust among users of medical services and, in particular, elderly users (Shareef et al., 2021). Elderly users distrust the functioning of these AI-based systems and of the lack of personalization and responsiveness to their individual needs (Xing et al., 2021).

A section of the population is resistant to change and prefers to continue to conduct activities in the same way they have traditionally done them. Kannan et al. (2020) state that one of the main reasons for the low use of AI in health care despite its potential is that people prefer to manage situations manually rather than using this new technology.

Ultimately, digital health care represents an opportunity to improve health care services, and it is possible that many of the innovations created to continue remote medical care during COVID-19 will continue to be employed subsequent to the end of the pandemic (Spanakis et al. 2021). Therefore, attention must be paid to the barriers posed by the digital divide in this area, and problems in accessing these services today must be addressed early, preventing disparities from continuing to widen.

In terms of education, the digital divide has also been an obstacle during the pandemic as digital platforms, some of them gamified and AI-based, have been used during this period to continue the distance learning process. In this context, students who do not have digital devices or internet connections, as well as those with few skills to cope in the digital world, have been disadvantaged. For example, Muflih et al. (2020) analyze the experience of university students in Jordan with online learning during the pandemic. Only 16.5 % of the participants in this study claimed to have been able to easily access the internet. In terms of the barriers they faced, students highlighted a lack of experience with online teaching tools (74.3 %) and limited technological expertise (75.1 %). Chakraborty et al. (2021) conducted a similar study in an Indian university and found that 66 % of the students who participated in it stated that online teaching makes them phobic about losing their internet connection.

Around the world, a number of initiatives have emerged to bridge this gap in education and facilitate the continuation of education through digital channels. These initiatives have mainly focused on the donation of digital devices to ensure access to online learning for all students. For example, in Hong Kong, used computers have been donated to underprivileged families, and assistance in paying for internet services has been provided (Shek, 2021). In Câmara de Lobos (Portugal), the authorities of the municipality created a Facebook campaign in April 2020 requesting the donation of computers with the aim of enabling all students in the locality to receive online education (Covid19People, 2020).

Another example is that of Cognita, an international group of schools that adopted Century, the AI-based gamified educational platform discussed in the previous chapter of this book. Cognita engaged Century's services as part of its transformation strategy to cope with the effects of COVID-19 and facilitate the continuation of the distance teaching-learning process. Now, since students need electronic devices to access Century, Cognita distributed more than 12000 laptops and tablets to its students so that they could enjoy this teaching method (Golding, 2021).

It is also worth noting that there are doubts about the effectiveness of the strategy of closing schools to curb the spread of COVID-19. As Silverman et al. (2020) argue, such interventions with significant adverse effects on a certain population group are justified if there is strong evidence that they offer benefits to another set of individuals. However, the closure of schools makes it difficult to continue the learning process, which is exacerbated by the digital divide; and evidence about the ability of school closures to slow the spread of the new coronavirus is limited. This leads to ethical debate about the appropriateness of this measure in the context of COVID-19 (Silverman et al., 2020). Joffe (2021) also notes the ineffectiveness of school and college closures in mitigating the increase in COVID-19 infections and the harms of this measure, such as increased disparities. Joffe (2021) and Silverman et al. (2020) advocate raising awareness among parents, students, and teachers of the low risk associated with face-to-face teaching and allowing a return to the classroom as soon as possible.

Ultimately, gamification and AI harbor great potential to mitigate the adverse effects of the pandemic in health care and education. However, those responsible for applications must be aware of the existence of the digital divide and the potential harm it can cause to the most vulnerable population. Therefore, progress in the development of technological innovations must be accompanied by solutions that allow access to these services despite not having the necessary resources such as digital devices or an adequate internet connection. Otherwise, some individuals will not be able to enjoy the benefits that these applications offer in health care and education. The main ethical challenge in this regard is the essential nature of both services.

5.3. Transparency

Transparency in the operation and in the terms and conditions of use of digital applications, including gamified and AI-based applications, represents an essential element for their ethical management (Raftopoulos, 2014; Walmsley, 2021). Transparency ensures that no user is harmed through the use of these systems, making it a feature of great importance for the generation of trust (Larsson and Heintz, 2020).

Referring to gamification, there is an ethical concern about the possibility of creating designs that lead to modifications in user behavior based on manipulation that would not otherwise occur (Goethe, 2020). A bad gamified design leads to unintended results. At best, gamification has no effect on users. Through this design, users are not motivated, and their behavior is not modified, rendering gamification ineffective (Zainuddin et al., 2020).

In the worst-case scenario, gamification negatively affects the motivation of individuals. Users of the gamified experience may think that it is all about rewards and punishments or believe that the social pressure to which they are subjected is excessive, which demotivates them and causes the opposite effect to the desired one (Mitchell et al., 2020). Collaborative creation from a multidisciplinary point of view facilitates the effectiveness of gamified experiences. In other words, researchers and gamification specialists should participate in its development together with professionals from the field in which the experience is framed. For example, a gamified health care application should be created by a group of gamification experts and health care professionals (Cuevas-Lara et al., 2021).

In the cases discussed above, it is assumed that gamification does not have a positive effect on user motivation due to design flaws that have occurred unintentionally. In other words, it is an error on the part of the designers that leads to a different result than expected. However, designers can also try to manipulate users through gamification and use deception and confusion to get them to perform certain behaviors that would not otherwise occur. In such a situation, those responsible for the experience establish dark patterns to confuse individuals (Goethe, 2020).

The intention of this manipulation may be to affect the well-being of the users. In such a case, we would be addressing paternalistic and educational designs that attempt to correct behaviors. The ethical problem that arises in this regard is the limitation of the freedom and autonomy of individuals, even if the design seeks to give them a benefit and improve their welfare (Tep et al., 2021).

However, designers may also seek to manipulate users to obtain a benefit of their own from the person responsible for the gamified experience. This sometimes occurs in the gamified activities created by companies as part of their marketing strategy to increase sales and thus revenues (Tep et al., 2021). The problem lies in the fact that the participants themselves may not be aware that techniques expressly devised to influence their behavior have been employed (Thorpe and Roper, 2019). All this has a negative impact on the transparency that gamified experiences must possess in order to meet the requirements posed by their ethical management, which are applicable to the COVID-19 context.

Regarding AI, there is a great deal of debate about the transparency of its operations and its ethical implications (Walmsley, 2021). This technology is based on complex systems that are difficult for the general population to understand. In addition, advances in AI research have led to the creation of models that offer more accurate predictions. However, this increase in accuracy is accompanied by increased model complexity (Linardatos et al., 2021). White box models, such as linear regressions and logistic regressions, also called glass box models, are inherently explainable models (Antoniadi et al., 2021). As a consequence of the increased complexity of AI-based systems, so-called black box models have emerged. Black box models are opaque and inherently inexplicable models whose internal learning processes are unknown (Antoniadi et al., 2021; Meske et al., 2020).

While black box models make more accurate predictions than white box models, their interpretation is more complex (Linardatos et al., 2021; Subudhi et al., 2020). Therefore, as Subudhi et al. (2020) state, decision-makers making decisions regarding the application of AI in a real-world environment must consider the risks and benefits of both types of models and assess the interpretability and accuracy of each to select the most appropriate model.

In some industries, there is widespread reliance on the predictions of black box models, and no explanation is required as to why the result has occurred. In these cases, such as in marketing, there are usually no direct consequences if the AI-based system fails. In other sectors, on the contrary, the critical nature of the decisions requires an explanation of the reasons on which the prediction is based (Burkart and Huber, 2021). The latter is the case in health care, where decisions affect the health of patients and may even be a decision between life and death. As a consequence, the black box represents one of the main challenges facing the application of AI in the health care sector (Mohammad Rahimi et al., 2021).

This phenomenon causes health care professionals to be unaware of what motives have led the algorithm to offer a certain diagnosis. This lack of explanation can cause mistrust and represent a barrier to its implementation. Therefore, these applications, in addition to improving health services, must be reliable and easy to understand (Antoniadi et al., 2021). For example, the diagnosis offered may be implausible if compared with the data held by a physician, generating suspicion about its performance. Moreover, if a practitioner distrusts the diagnosis, it is unlikely that a patient will trust it (Kasperbauer, 2021; Watson et al., 2019). Therefore, when AI is used in health services, a clinician must understand the results that the algorithm yields and, through communication with the patient, assess the diagnosis and make appropriate decisions (Kolanska et al., 2021).

Medical professionals may also be wary of AI-based diagnostic health systems if their training has been conducted using data from a sample belonging to a certain population group (Murphy et al., 2021). If this occurs, the particularities of other population sectors are not being contemplated by the system, leading to erroneous predictions. Therefore, it is understandable that some health care professionals are critical of certain clinical applications based on AI and reject them if they have not been trained in a broader context.

One of the main applications of AI in the health care setting during the pandemic has been the diagnosis of COVID-19 from clinical image analysis. However, an AI-based system may fail and give an erroneous result. In such a case, a patient who actually has COVID-19 may not be diagnosed with

COVID-19; therefore, necessary precautions such as isolation may not be taken, and treatment of the disease may not be initiated in its initial period. In such a situation, the ethical dilemma arises as to who is responsible for the diagnosis if it has been offered by an algorithm. Neri et al. (2020a) argue that the physician is responsible for the diagnosis when it has been elaborated by IA and that physicians should know how the AI-based systems they employ work and should assume the associated risk.

Ishmaev et al. (2021) assert that the effectiveness and suitability of AI-based COVID-19 diagnostic systems need to be analyzed before they are employed on a large scale to avoid the serious consequences of diagnostic errors. Furthermore, they reject that this new technology will replace the judgment of health care professionals in the short term. Some medical societies have taken a position on its use during the pandemic. For example, the Italian Society of Medical and Interventional Radiology supports research into the use of AI to predict and forecast the evolution of the disease caused by the new coronavirus. However, they do not support the use of AI in this context for diagnosis and emphasize that this technology should not replace other diagnostic tests that have been proven to be effective (Neri et al., 2020b).

For all these reasons, the adoption of AI in different sectors, including health care, is conditioned by the explainability of its predictions (Confalonieri et al., 2021). Lack of knowledge about how AI works and why it makes predictions and decisions generates mistrust and ethical concerns among users, which negatively affects the practical use of AI-based applications. As a consequence, in recent years, there has been a resurgence of interest in explainable artificial intelligence (XAI), an area of research that emerged more than three decades ago (Miller, 2019).

This explainability refers to post hoc explainability, which is obtained by means of different techniques that convert an uninterpretable model into an explainable model (Barriedo Arrieta et al., 2020). These post hoc techniques are applied after the algorithm has been trained (Alves et al., 2021). It should be clarified that post hoc explanations are required by black box models since, unlike white box models, they are not inherently explainable (Antoniadi et al., 2021). Markus et al. (2021, p.2) define explainability as follows: "An AI system is explainable if the task model is intrinsically interpretable (here the AI system is the task model) or if the noninterpretable task model is complemented with an interpretable and faithful explanation (here the AI system also contains a post hoc explanation)".

The explainability of a black box model can be global or local (Petch et al., 2021). Global explainability refers to the explanation of the overall functioning of the model. Global explainability is key during the model development phase, during which it is verified that the learning of the algorithm is proceeding properly and yields consistent predictions. Local explainability, conversely, refers to the explanation of a specific prediction. That is, local explainability informs us about the reasons why a model has made a certain decision, which is related to an improvement in the transparency of AI-based applications (Petch et al., 2021).

In the health care domain, local explainability represents the explanation of the reasons why an AI-based system delivers a particular outcome such as, for example, a diagnosis or prognosis. In the context of COVID-19, and especially during the first months of the pandemic, AI-based systems can be of great help in guiding health care professionals in making decisions in the environment of uncertainty caused by the lack of knowledge about the behavior of the new coronavirus. For example, Pan et al. (2020) develop a model that, through AI, predicts the risk of COVID-19 patients in an intensive care unit. To address the black box, they employ techniques that provide local explainability. In this way, the model, in addition to predicting the prognosis, explains the prediction in a reasonable way. This makes it easier for users to trust the results (Pan et al., 2020).

For all these reasons, transparency is a key element in the ethical analysis of AI-based gamified systems used during the pandemic. This is particularly relevant to AI and, in particular, to the black box problem. As discussed, black box models make more accurate predictions, which facilitates the development of more effective applications to fight COVID-19 in different areas. However, black box models are inherently inexplicable. Their inexplicability, while it can be addressed through XAI, is an obstacle to their practical application. This is particularly relevant in the health care domain, where although AI-based systems are being developed to diagnose and forecast COVID-19, their application in real-world settings is almost nil.

Finally, it should be noted that AI-based applications have been employed during the pandemic despite their low transparency. One example is Health Code, a Chinese tracking app that assesses the contagion risk of individuals through an algorithm (Liang, 2020). Health Code assesses factors such as travel history and contact with people who may be infected and, based on these data, provides a QR code to each user that can be one of three colors: green, yellow and red. This color indicates the possibility of contagion. If the QR code is green, the individual has a low risk and can move freely. However, yellow and red colors indicate medium and high risks of infection, respectively, which imply the need for home confinement to prevent the spread of the virus (Liang, 2020).

Presenting a green code in Health Code is a mandatory requirement to access public places in more than 300 Chinese cities. Some of the places affected by this measure are schools, restaurants and public transportation (Liang, 2020). In contrast, a yellow or red code can mean the isolation of the individual for a period between 7 and 14 days (Mozur et al., 2020).

The problem arises from the lack of knowledge of what data this application shares with the Chinese authorities and how exactly the application works since it has not been explained how this color classification is elaborated. All this has generated fear and bewilderment among the Chinese population who must comply with home confinement if the app gives them a yellow or red code, even if they do not know the reasons (Mozur et al., 2020).

Zhou et al. (2021b) analyze opinions of health and public safety experts and the general population about this app. To do so, they interview several of these experts and conduct a public survey. The most recurring theme in the interviews with health and public safety experts was privacy. Specifically, the experts indicated that they did not know how long the app developers were going to keep their personal data and were concerned about this. As for the general population, only 18 of the 148 individuals who participated in the survey stated that the app caused them an inconvenience. Among the drawbacks stated, experts were concerned about privacy. The protection of privacy in data processing is an issue that also concerns ethics in these systems. Therefore, their gamification and AI during the pandemic are discussed below and analyzed from the point of view of ethics.

5.4. Privacy

Advancing knowledge about the new coronavirus and discovering which strategies are most effective in fighting the pandemic requires access to information that is amenable to analysis. These data can come from numerous sources, such as public databases and websites (Abd-Alrazaq et al., 2020). This pandemic, unlike previous pandemics such as the Spanish flu in 1918 and the Asian flu in 1957, occurred in a period characterized by digitization and connectivity that makes it easier to obtain data to combat the virus (Sharma and Bashir, 2020). Data sharing is essential for the research and development of responses capable of handling COVID-19 (Lenert and McSwain, 2020).

However, ethics about individual privacy and regulations about data protection restrain possibilities in this regard. Generally, two approaches to data and data privacy are identified in the context of COVID-19: data-first and privacy-first approaches (Fahey and Hino, 2020). The data-first approach advocates allowing access to data for researchers and authorities responsible for pandemic measures. Under the privacy-first approach, by contrast, privacy protection takes precedence, and each individual is given control over his or her data (Fahey and Hino, 2020). The following are some of the limitations faced by gamification and AI in the pandemic context with reference to data collection and the protection of the population's privacy.

Regarding gamification, Mavroeidi et al. (2019) analyze the relationship of several of its elements (points, roles and avatars, among others) with the main privacy requirements to study the degree to which gamified experiences protect the privacy of their users. The privacy requirements on which they focus their analysis are anonymity, pseudonymity, unlinkability, undetectability and unobservability. First, Mavroeidi et al. (2019) highlight the risk involved in the mandatory creation of profiles in order to access a gamified application. It is usual to create profiles by registering an email account or an account on a social network such as Facebook. Linking the virtual identity used to operate the gamified application with the identity on other platforms facilitates data registration and jeopardizes users' privacy.

For example, if the gamified experience includes challenges within its design, users can discover the identity of their opponents and access their personal information. In such a case, the anonymity and unlinkability of the participants is not protected. Moreover, other elements of gamification, such as teams, are likely to violate all privacy principles (anonymity, pseudonymity, unlinkability, undetectability and unobservability). Elements that enable communication between users put their privacy at risk by establishing the possibility of revealing data about their identity, even if no prior profile has been created and linked to an email account or a social network (Mavroeidi et al., 2019).

These risks to privacy protection are found in all areas of gamification application, including health care and education. Some researchers have shown interest in analyzing individuals' perception of privacy in gamified systems in these two sectors. For example, Yang and Li (2021b) study how various gamification features influence two stressors, privacy invasion and social overload, in gamified health care applications. These authors conclude that competition and interactivity are positively related to both stressors. In other words, competition and interactivity in gamified applications are seen by users as elements that invade their privacy and cause social overload.

A priori, one might think that this invasion of privacy implies a lower intention to participate in a gamified experience. However, this is not always the case. Proof of this is the study by Aguiar-Castillo et al. (2020), which yields surprising results in this regard. According to the results of their analysis, the loss of privacy does not harm university students' intention to use an educational gamified application. Moreover, the loss of privacy is positively related to their intention to use it.

Aguiar-Castillo et al. (2020) argue that the gains participants obtain through their participation in the gamified experience, such as achieving a higher score, may outweigh the risk this poses to their privacy. Therefore, they conclude that while there is evidence that loss of privacy negatively affects technology adoption, their study shows that these effects depend on the application context and user characteristics. In particular, the intention to use a gamified application by university students does not seem to decrease as a consequence of the potential loss of privacy.

In short, gamification poses a risk to users' privacy protection both generally and in the context of the pandemic. This poses a problem for its use from an ethical point of view. However, individuals, as in the study conducted by Aguiar-Castillo et al. (2020), may decide to use a gamified application despite this risk if it provides them a benefit that justifies the risk. This could occur in the case of gamified applications created in the framework of the pandemic that seek to mitigate the effects of COVID-19, given that they offer a clear benefit to their users.

With regard to AI, and as discussed in Chapter 3 of this book, a large volume of data is needed to train an AI-based system and get it to work properly. In the pandemic context, the problem emerges from the paucity of existing data in this regard and the difficulty of obtaining it without harming patient privacy. For example, developing an AI-based application capable of detecting that a patient has COVID-19 from clinical images requires gathering a large set of clinical images with which to train the prediction algorithm. However, the availability of repositories of such images is very limited. This is because in order to use these resources in scientific research, the consent of the patients from whom the images have been obtained must be requested beforehand since the information is confidential (López-Cabrera et al., 2021).

Regarding AI-based COVID-19 tracking applications, Bengio et al. (2020) state that those responsible for these applications must request explicit consent from users for their data to be used in algorithm training. This consent must be clearly requested. In other words, those responsible for tracking applications must not hide the request for this permission within a lengthy text establishing all the terms of their privacy policy, but rather must do so in a transparent manner. This ensures that the users agree to the release of their information.

Pickering (2021) also state that consent to data transfer when downloading a mobile app may be insufficient. In addition, Pickering highlights the possibility that an individual may not continue to use an app because he or she has lost trust in it and fears that its use will harm his or her privacy. Therefore, Pickering (2021) recommends that those responsible for mobile applications remain vigilant and seek to identify their users' concerns about the protection of their data. In addition, Pickering adds that those responsible for these apps should also take care of their public image and demonstrate their integrity on an ongoing basis to encourage user engagement. These arguments given by Bengio et al. (2020) and Pickering (2021) could be applied to all applications created during the pandemic to fight COVID-19, not only those dedicated to contact tracing.

Moreover, those responsible for AI-based COVID-19 tracking applications must protect the privacy of users who have consented to have their information used to train algorithms. Therefore, the data used should not contain sufficient details to allow identification of the individuals to whom they belong if these data are correlated with data from other sources. Aggregating and anonymizing the data with which an algorithm is trained makes it difficult to reveal the identity of an individual when crossing this information with other available datasets that also include data on the subject in question (Cortés et al., 2021). Specifically, data are considered anonymous if it is impossible to reidentify individuals in a reasonably practical way (Hedlund et al., 2020). This facilitates the protection of the privacy of individuals who provide their data.

Another possible solution to protect the privacy of user data is federated learning (FL). As discussed in Chapter 3 of this book, the training of algorithms in FL occurs in a decentralized manner across multiple devices. That is, FL does not require the collection and storage of a large dataset on a single server or infrastructure, which helps to improve privacy protection (Aledhari et al., 2020).

FL can be of great help in advancing clinical research about COVID-19 as it facilitates privacy protection of sensitive data such as health-related data. Practically, FL has been employed for the diagnosis of COVID-19 through clinical imaging and for the prediction of the mortality of COVID-19 patients (Qian and Zhang, 2021). However, it should be noted that it has some drawbacks compared to other IA systems, such as its high data communication costs and the detrimental effect of data heterogeneity on the performance of the FL algorithm (Zhang et al., 2021c).

Health data are of great utility to train and feed AI-based systems in the context of pandemics and can greatly help in research on COVID-19. However, this is sensitive information as it is related to the health of individuals and thus their privacy. In this context, the dilemma arises between the rights of individuals to decide not to cede their information to institutions and research entities and the potential benefits that these data can offer to society as a whole. Larson et al. (2020) advocate anonymizing and aggregating clinical data and treating them as a public good given the interest they hold in research and health service improvement. Other authors such as Dagliati et al. (2021) and Dron et al. (2021) also highlight the importance of sharing these data to facilitate the development of pandemic research.

Another problem emerges when personal information given up to fuel AI-based systems focused on mitigating the effects of COVID-19 is employed for perverse purposes such as marketing (Chen and See, 2020). Likewise, there is some concern about the future of AI-based tracking and surveillance technologies employed to contain the spread of the new coronavirus, which could become standard practice within government public health strategies when the pandemic has ended (Kiliç, 2021). Another related fear is the possibility that governments will take advantage of the special circumstances surrounding the pandemic and use the data obtained in the context of COVID-19 for other purposes when this period is over (Naudé, 2020).

In conclusion, privacy protection is a major area of importance within ethics that may pose a barrier to the development and application of AI-based gamified systems during the pandemic. Data collection and processing are essential to the operations of these applications. However, this practice puts the privacy of individuals at risk. Moreover, the relevance of privacy protection is that there are different regulations around the world that regulate the use of personal data. Some of these regulations and their implications during COVID-19 are outlined below.

5.5. Legal issues

Given all these arguments in favor of taking care of ethics in systems based on gamification and AI developed in the context of the pandemic, one might think that greater attention to ethics is related to greater acceptance and participation through these applications on the part of the population. However, this does not necessarily need to be the case. Proof of this is the study by El-Haddadeh et al. (2021), which provides surprising results in this regard.

El-Haddadeh et al. (2021) analyze the ethical care and effectiveness achieved by two AI-based proximity tracking and tracing apps created in two different countries to curb the spread of COVID-19. Specifically, they focus their study on Qatar's EHTERAZ app and the UK NHS COVID-19 app. As a result, they find that Qatar's EHTERAZ app, despite performing poorer in terms of ethical management, has made a significant contribution to containing the pandemic. The UK NHS COVID-19 app, however, takes better care of ethical concerns but has had little success in its territory. El-Haddadeh et al. (2021) attribute this divergence between the impact and the degree of compliance with the ethical framework to the different capacities of the governments of each of these countries to enforce the use of the apps. The UK has a more limited ability as it must comply with stricter data protection regulations than Qatar (El-Haddadeh et al., 2021).

The mandatory or voluntary nature of COVID-19 tracking apps is a controversial issue (Lalmuanawma et al., 2020). In the pandemic context, the AI-based systems used must offer a public benefit that justifies the associated ethical risks (Gasser et al., 2020). Moreover, this decision is conditioned by the regulations in force in each country, and each territory has different regulations in this regard.

Therefore, the ability to apply AI-based systems to combat COVID-19 varies between countries and regions. These circumstances require a specific analysis to identify the real possibilities of implementation and what requirements must be respected according to the regulations in force in each territory. For example, Almada and Maranhão (2021) study the ethical and legal challenges faced by COVID-19 diagnostic apps using AI and voice recordings in Brazil. To do so, they rely on the requirements imposed by Brazil's General Data Protection Law. Ekong et al. (2020) analyze the possibility of implementing digital contact tracing apps in the context delimited by the National Data Protection Regulation of Nigeria.

One of the strictest regulations is the General Data Protection Regulation (GDPR) of the European Union. With regard to clinical data, the GDPR states that each individual controls his or her own sensitive data and must give explicit consent to its use or sharing. That is, information such as clinical images, which represent a great opportunity to create COVID-19 diagnostic systems, is owned by patients. In order for these data to be used for algorithm training, patients must give their consent (Brady and Neri, 2020). Moreover, the GDPR reflects the importance of XAI in recent times as this regulation requires organizations employing AI to provide explanations as to why an algorithm arrives at a particular decision (Payrovnaziri et al., 2020).

The truth is that the COVID-19 pandemic has been an unprecedented worldwide crisis, generating uncertainty about the limits of action in such circumstances from a legal point of view. In March 2020, at the onset of the pandemic, data protection authorities in Italy, the European country most affected by COVID-19 at the time, warned of the possibility of infringing on the privacy of the population through the collection and use of data with the aim of mitigating the spread of the new coronavirus by noninstitutional actors (Ienca and Vayena, 2020).

Shortly thereafter, the European Data Protection Board noted the importance of data protection in the context of COVID-19 and stated that the GDPR permits the processing of personal data in health emergencies if it is done proportionately, in the public interest, and without harming the rights and freedoms of each individual (Ienca and Vayena, 2020).

In the United States, the Health Insurance Portability and Accountability Act (HIPAA) restricts the use of identifiable health data on the grounds of the harm that its use may cause to the dignity of patients (Krass et al., 2021). However, during the pandemic, the Office of Civil Rights at the U.S. Department of Health and Human Services clarified some of the terms relevant to privacy protection and the sharing of medical information in the emergency context of COVID-19 (Hoffman, 2020).

Specifically, the Office of Civil Rights stated that the HIPAA permits the sharing of information without patient consent if this is necessary to treat the patient himself or herself or another subject. As Hoffman (2020) states, with regard to COVID-19, having a vast pool of medical information can facilitate the treatment of other patients. In addition, the Office of Civil Rights also clarified that the HIPAA allows covered entities to transfer data to public health authorities and law enforcement without patient consent (Hoffman, 2020). Additionally, it should be noted that the HIPAA privacy regulation applies to health care-related entities. Thus, during the pandemic, various nonhealth care-related entities have extracted personal data without patient consent for the purpose of selling it to third-party agents such as marketers and insurers (van Assen et al., 2020).

However, there are countries and regions with less stringent data protection regulations. In these cases, the benefit of society takes precedence over individual rights. There are also cases in which the ownership of clinical data does not lie with the patient but with the health care facility performing the analyses (Brady and Neri, 2020). These differences may hinder the development of research on the use of AI against COVID-19 in territories whose regulations offer greater protection to patients because they make it more difficult to obtain data (Brady and Neri, 2020).

A special case is South Korea. South Korea's Personal Information Protection Act (PIPA) dates to 2011 and prohibits the collection and use of personal data without the consent of individuals (Ryan, 2020). However, this country was severely affected by MERS, a syndrome caused by another coronavirus, in 2015. At that time, the PIPA was identified as an obstacle to curbing the spread of the virus. For this reason, the regulation about the use of personal data during health emergencies was changed in Korea, which has been helpful in containing the transmission of COVID-19 in this country (Ryan, 2020). This example shows the importance of having experience in a given circumstance, which has led to exceptions being made at specific times if the collective benefit to be obtained is much greater than the individual harm.

Ultimately, the ability to implement AI-based gamified systems to address the pandemic is conditioned by legal restrictions on the collection and use of personal data. These privacy protection regulations are closely related to ethics. They aim to protect the rights of individuals and pay particular attention to clinical data. Clinical data are essential for the development and application of algorithms in the context of COVID-19, but they are sensitive data whose privacy must be protected. Privacy is also one of the areas that encompasses ethics. Therefore, the analysis of the ethical plane of AI-based gamified applications during the pandemic must consider the regulations regarding data protection and privacy in force in each country.

6. Conclusions and final reflections

The aim of this book is to analyze the use of gamification and AI in the health and educational fields during the pandemic. To this end, a review of the main applications of gamification and AI during this period has been carried out, as well as an analysis of four cases in which both gamification and AI are combined and their usefulness in the context characterized by COVID-19. The main conclusions reached through this work and some final reflections are presented below.

First, gamification has been used in both the health care and educational fields. In the health care field, gamification has been introduced in apps dedicated to *patient management* and physical activity. This technique has also been used in campaigns to raise awareness and prevent the spread of COVID-19. In some cases, it has been of great help in motivating users, but in others, on the contrary, it seems to have had no effect. For example, the introduction of gamification in NZ COVID Tracer, the New Zealand Ministry of Health's contact tracing app, did not increase the volume of engagement on the platform (Chen, 2021b). However, no studies have analyzed the reasons for this lack of success. In terms of education, gamification appears to have motivated students and encouraged their engagement at a time of uncertainty when their mental health, ability to concentrate and academic performance have been affected (Kecojevic et al., 2020).

Second, a large number of applications have been developed within the context of COVID-19 based on AI, although their relevance has not been as high as expected. These applications are divided into several areas: prediction and surveillance, *patient management*, disease diagnosis and prognosis, and drug and vaccine research. Although AI seemed to have greater potential than it has actually had to combat the pandemic (Naudé, 2020), the truth is that some projects based on it have been successful. An example of a successful application of AI in this context is chatbots that resolve doubts about the situation, prevention and management of the disease caused by the new coronavirus. In terms of education, most of the AI-based applications used during COVID-19 have been platforms that had been created previously. That is, during the pandemic, AI-based systems have been developed to mitigate the effects of COVID-19 in the health domain. In the educational domain, on the other hand, preexisting platforms have been used to solve the challenge posed by the transfer to distance education.

The limited scope of AI-based applications created during this period in the health care field and the lack of application development in the educational field may be due to the cost and time required to build these systems, as well as the need for large datasets to work properly. It is also worth noting the great usefulness that AI has shown to curb the dissemination of *misinformation through* social networks. Platforms such as Facebook and Twitter have made use of it to detect false information, protecting the population from behaviors that, based on this *misinformation,* can threaten their own health and that of others.

Third, the analysis of the four cases in which gamification and AI are combined shows that the combination of the two has been a significant help during this period. Both DreamLab: Corona-AI and uMore in the health care field and Century and ELSA Speak in the educational field have facilitated adaptation to the new circumstances or have accelerated the return to normality through gamification and AI. However, it seems that during this period, no gamified applications based on AI have been developed within the educational field, as has happened with those that do not integrate a gamified design in this same sector. Century and ELSA Speak, the two applications analyzed in the fourth chapter, were created years before the pandemic.

The reason for this can be found, again, in the cost and time required to build these systems, as well as the need for large datasets to function properly. In the early stages of the pandemic, quick solutions were needed to transfer learning to the digital medium. It makes no sense to spend the effort to create new applications and train the algorithms on which they are based if preexisting applications that offer these services, such as Century and ELSA Speak, are already available. In the health field, on the other hand, new applications have been developed in the context of COVID-19, such as uMore, and projects aimed at the new coronavirus have been launched through preexisting platforms, such as the Corona-AI project within DreamLab.

Finally, it is worth noting a major barrier faced by this type of digital solution – the *digital divide.* Not being able to access digital health services because one does not have an internet connection or does not know how to operate electronic devices can increase the digital divide and harm the most vulnerable population groups (Ramsetty and Adams, 2020). In terms of education, families with fewer resources may not have a device with an internet connection at home for the student to access the educational platform. Additionally, some students are not prepared for this transfer of education to the digital realm and lack the necessary skills to cope with it. In such a case, they will depend on other family members to set up and connect to the educational platform (Iivari et al., 2020). This issue should be considered during the development and implementation of these applications to carry out measures that disadvantage some groups of the population.

Other ethical aspects to be taken into account are transparency in the operation of these applications and the protection of users' privacy. These aspects mainly affect IA and the healthcare field. On the one hand, the complexity of AI makes it difficult to know the reasons why the system produces a prediction. This lack of knowledge can affect its application in real environments. AI-based diagnostic and prognostic systems can help healthcare professionals in decision-making. However, if the clinician does not know why the system predicts an outcome, it is likely to be unreliable.

Concerning user privacy, an ethical dilemma arises in the context of the pandemic between protecting personal data privacy or allowing the authorities responsible for managing the situation to access it to investigate and take appropriate action. In particular, data privacy protection represents an obstacle to the development of AI-based systems since algorithms need a large amount of data to be trained and function properly. This ethical dilemma is especially relevant in the healthcare sector. Mitigating the spread of COVID-19 and treating patients using AI requires access to a large set of clinical data. Therefore, the question must be asked whether, in these exceptional circumstances of a health emergency, the potential benefit to society at large or the protection of the privacy of each individual takes precedence.

Acknowledgments

Project co-financed by the European Regional Development Fund (80 %) and the Regional Government of Extremadura (file GR18123).

Proyecto cofinanciado por el Fondo Europeo de Desarrollo Regional (80 %) y la Junta de Extremadura (expediente GR18123).

References

1MillionBot. (2021a). *Hi, I'm Carina*. Retrieved from https://1millionbot. com/chatbot-coronavirus/ [accessed 31/08/2021].

1MillionBot. (2021b). *Meet Carina*. Retrieved from https://1millionbot. com/chatbot-coronavirus-info/ [accessed 31/08/2021].

Abd-Alrazaq, A., Alajlani, M., Alhuwail, D., Schneider, J., Al-Kuwari, S., Shah, Z., Hamdi, M., & Househ, M. (2020). Artificial intelligence in the fight against COVID-19: Scoping review. *Journal of Medical Internet Research*, 22(12), e20756.

Abdulkareem, M., & Petersen, S. E. (2021). The promise of AI in detection, diagnosis, and epidemiology for combating COVID-19: Beyond the hype. *Frontiers in Artificial Intelligence*, 4, 652669.

Aggarwal, D., Mittal, S., & Bali, V. (2021). Significance of non-academic parameters for predicting student performance using ensemble learning techniques. *International Journal of System Dynamics Applications (IJSDA)*, 10(3), 38–49.

Aguiar-Castillo, L., Hernández-López, L., De Saá-Pérez, P., & Pérez-Jiménez, R. (2020). Gamification as a motivation strategy for higher education students in tourism face-to-face learning. *Journal of Hospitality, Leisure, Sport & Tourism Education*, 27, 100267.

Ahmed, F. R. A., Ahmed, T. E., Saeed, R. A., Alhumyani, H., Abdel-Khalek, S., & Abu-Zinadah, H. (2021). Analysis and challenges of robust E-exams performance under COVID-19. *Results in Physics*, 23, 103987.

Ahuja, A. S., Reddy, V. P., & Marques, O. (2020). Artificial intelligence and COVID-19: A multidisciplinary approach. *Integrative Medicine Research*, 9(3), 100434.

Akour, I., Alshurideh, M., Al Kurdi, B., Al Ali, A., & Salloum, S. (2021). Using machine learning algorithms to predict people's intention to use mobile learning platforms during the COVID-19 pandemic: Machine learning approach. *JMIR Medical Education*, 7(1), e24032.

Al-Qaness, M. A., Ewees, A. A., Fan, H., & Abd El Aziz, M. (2020). Optimization method for forecasting confirmed cases of COVID-19 in China. *Journal of Clinical Medicine*, 9(3), 674.

Aledhari, M., Razzak, R., Parizi, R. M., & Saeed, F. (2020). Federated learning: A survey on enabling technologies, protocols, and applications. *IEEE Access*, *8*, 140699–140725.

Allam, Z. (2020). The first 50 days of COVID-19: A detailed chronological timeline and extensive review of literature documenting the pandemic. *Surveying the Covid-19 Pandemic and Its Implications*, 1–7.

Allam, Z., Dey, G., & Jones, D. S. (2020). Artificial intelligence (AI) provided early detection of the coronavirus (COVID-19) in China and will influence future Urban health policy internationally. *AI*, *1*(2), 156–165.

Almada, M., & Maranhão, J. (2021). Voice-based diagnosis of covid-19: Ethical and legal challenges. *International Data Privacy Law*. In Press.

Almalki, M., & Giannicchi, A. (2021). Health apps for combating COVID-19: Descriptive review and taxonomy. *JMIR mHealth and uHealth*, *9*(3), e24322.

Almufty, H. B., Mohammed, S. A., Abdullah, A. M., & Merza, M. A. (2021). Potential adverse effects of COVID19 vaccines among Iraqi population; a comparison between the three available vaccines in Iraq; a retrospective cross-sectional study. *Diabetes & Metabolic Syndrome: Clinical Research & Reviews*, *15*(5), 102207.

Alsamawi, F. N., & Kurnaz, S. (2021). A framework for adopting gamified learning systems in smart schools during COVID-19. *Applied Nanoscience*. In Press.

Alves, M. A., Castro, G. Z., Oliveira, B. A. S., Ferreira, L. A., Ramírez, J. A., Silva, R., & Guimarães, F. G. (2021). Explaining machine learning based diagnosis of COVID-19 from routine blood tests with decision trees and criteria graphs. *Computers in Biology and Medicine*, *132*, 104335.

Amazon. (June 1, 2020). *Alexa and Amazon Devices COVID-19 resources.* Retrieved from https://www.aboutamazon.com/news/devices/alexa-and-amazon-devices-covid-19-resources [accessed 08/25/2021].

Anderson, C., Bieck, C., & Marshall, A. (2021). How business is adapting to COVID-19: Executive insights reveal post-pandemic opportunities. *Strategy & Leadership*, *49*(1), 38–47.

Anderson, J. (March 5, 2020). *With 290 million kids out of school, coronavirus is putting online learning to the test.* Quartz. Retrieved from https://qz.com/1812638/millions-of-kids-testing-e-learning-after-coronavirus-school-closures/ [accessed 11/09/2021].

Antoniadi, A. M., Du, Y., Guendouz, Y., Wei, L., Mazo, C., Becker, B. A., & Mooney, C. (2021). Current challenges and future opportunities for XAI in machine learning-based clinical decision support systems: A systematic review. *Applied Sciences*, *11*(11), 5088.

Araújo, R. L., da Silva Sena, T., & Endo, P. T. (2021). Gamification applied to an elderly monitoring system during the COVID-19 pandemic. *IEEE Latin America Transactions*, *19*(6), 1074–1082.

Areed, M. F., Amasha, M. A., Abougalala, R. A., Alkhalaf, S., & Khairy, D. (2021). Developing gamification e-quizzes based on an android app: The impact of asynchronous form. *Education and Information Technologies*, *26*, 4857–4878.

Arora, A., & Arora, A. (2020). Ethics in the age of COVID-19. *Internal and Emergency Medicine*, *15*, 889–890.

Asakura, K., Occhiuto, K., Todd, S., Leithead, C., & Clapperton, R. (2020). A call to action on artificial intelligence and social work education: Lessons learned from a simulation project using natural language processing. *Journal of Teaching in Social Work*, *40*(5), 501–518.

Baeza, C. (May 26, 2020). *BBVA employee online training, augmented during shelter in place*. BBVA. Retrieved from https://www.bbva.com/en/bbva-employee-online-training-augmented-during-shelter-in-place/ [accessed 31/08/2021].

Baeza, C. (29 April 2021). *Reskilling: BBVA trains its employees in new strategic skills*. BBVA. Retrieved from https://www.bbva.com/en/reskilling-bbva-trains-its-employees-in-new-strategic-skills/ [accessed 31/08/2021].

Banava, S., Jorquera, J., & Iyer, P. (2021). Virtual caries risk assessment workshop in COVID-19 era: Innovative game-based strategy. *Journal of Dental Education*. In Press.

Bansal, A., Padappayil, R. P., Garg, C., Singal, A., Gupta, M., & Klein, A. (2020). Utility of artificial intelligence amidst the COVID 19 pandemic: A review. *Journal of Medical Systems*, *44*, 156.

Barnawi, A., Chhikara, P., Tekchandani, R., Kumar, N., & Alzahrani, B. (2021). Artificial intelligence-enabled Internet of Things-based system for COVID-19 screening using aerial thermal imaging. *Future Generation Computer Systems, 124,* 119–132.

Barriedo Arrieta, A., Díaz-Rodríguez, N., Del Ser, J., Bennetot, A., Tabik, S., Barbado, A., ... & Herrera, F. (2020). Explainable Artificial Intelligence (XAI): Concepts, taxonomies, opportunities and challenges toward responsible AI. *Information Fusion, 58,* 82–115.

Bates, T., Cobo, C., Mariño, O., & Wheeler, S. (2020). Can artificial intelligence transform higher education? *International Journal of Educational Technology in Higher Education, 17,* 42.

Bengio, Y., Janda, R., Yu, Y. W., Ippolito, D., Jarvie, M., Pilat, D., ... & Sharma, A. (2020). The need for privacy with public digital contact tracing during the COVID-19 pandemic. *The Lancet Digital Health, 2*(7), e342–e344.

Benjumea, S. (May 18, 2021). *Telemedicine, mental health or wellness for the elderly. These are the startups selected for Google for Startups' 'Growth Academy: Health & WellBeing' in Madrid.* Google. Retrieved from https://espana.googleblog.com/2021/05/telemedicina-salud-mental-o-bienestar.html [accessed 07/09/2021].

Bilen, E., & Matros, A. (2021). Online cheating amid COVID-19. *Journal of Economic Behavior & Organization, 182,* 196–211.

Bitrián, P., Buil, I., & Catalán, S. (2021). Enhancing user engagement: The role of gamification in mobile apps. *Journal of Business Research, 132,* 170–185.

BlueDot. (n.d.). Retrieved from https://bluedot.global [accessed 31/08/2021].

Bogoch, I. I., Watts, A., Thomas-Bachli, A., Huber, C., Kraemer, M. U., & Khan, K. (2020). Pneumonia of unknown aetiology in Wuhan, China: Potential for international spread via commercial air travel. *Journal of Travel Medicine, 27*(2), taaa008.

Borzenkova, G., Golovátina-Mora, P., Ramirez, P. A. Z., & Sarmiento, J. M. H. (2021). Gamification Design for Behavior Change of Indigenous Communities in Choco, Colombia, During COVID-19 Pandemic. In: Spanellis, A., Harviainen, J. T. (Eds.), *Transforming Society and Organizations through Gamification* (pp. 309–334). Palgrave Macmillan, Cham.

Bouchareb, Y., Khaniabadi, P. M., Al Kindi, F., Al Dhuhli, H., Shiri, I., Zaidi, H., & Rahmim, A. (2021). Artificial intelligence-driven assessment of radiological images for COVID-19. *Computers in Biology and Medicine*, *136*, 104665.

Bowles, J. (March 10, 2020). *How Canadian AI start-up BlueDot spotted Coronavirus before anyone else had a clue*. Diginomica. Retrieved from https://diginomica.com/how-canadian-ai-start-bluedot-spotted-coronavi rus-anyone-else-had-clue [accessed 31/08/2021].

Bozkurt, A., Karadeniz, A., Baneres, D., Guerrero-Roldán, A. E., & Rodríguez, M. E. (2021). Artificial intelligence and reflections from educational landscape: A review of AI studies in half a century. *Sustainability*, *13*, 800.

Brady, A. P., & Neri, E. (2020). Artificial intelligence in radiology—ethical considerations. *Diagnostics*, *10*(4), 231.

Buheji, M. (2020). Fluid thinking for ageing parents-compensating the psychological risks of COVID-19 pandemic using gamification. *International Journal of Psychology and Behavioral Sciences*, *10*(4), 93–99.

Burkart, N., & Huber, M. F. (2021). A survey on the explainability of supervised machine learning. *Journal of Artificial Intelligence Research*, *70*, 245–317.

Cao, J., Yang, T., Lai, I. K. W., & Wu, J. (2021). Student acceptance of intelligent tutoring systems during COVID-19: The effect of political influence. *The International Journal of Electrical Engineering & Education*. In Press.

Century. (May 20, 2020). *Lebanon adopts CENTURY to sustain learning throughout school closures*. Retrieved from https://www.century.tech/news/lebanon-adopts-century-to-sustain-learning-throughout-school-closures/ [accessed 11/09/2021].

Century. (2021a). Retrieved from https://www.century.tech [accessed 11/09/2021].

Century. (2021b). *Our impact*. Retrieved from https://www.century.tech/our-impact/ [accessed 11/09/2021].

Century. (January 18, 2021c). *How Eton College uses technology to bolster traditional teaching*. Retrieved from https://www.century.tech/news/how-eton-college-uses-technology-to-bolster-traditional-teaching/ [accessed11/09/2021].

Chakraborty, P., Mittal, P., Gupta, M. S., Yadav, S., & Arora, A. (2021). Opinion of students on online education during the COVID- 19 pandemic. *Human Behavior and Emerging Technologies, 3*(3), 357–365.

Chassagnon, G., Vakalopoulou, M., Battistella, E., Christodoulidis, S., Hoang-Thi, T. N., Dangeard, S., ... & Paragios, N. (2021). AI-driven quantification, staging and outcome prediction of COVID-19 pneumonia. *Medical Image Analysis, 67,* 101860.

Chen, A. (April 12, 2021a). *The Contact Tracer app just got gamified. Here's what that means for you.* The Spinoff. Retrieved from https://the spinoff.co.nz/science/12-04-2021/the-contact-tracer-app-just-got-gamif ied-heres-what-that-means-for-you/ [accessed 27/08/2021].

Chen, A. (May 19, 2021b). *Lessons from our Covid tracing app.* Ideasroom. Retrieved from https://www.newsroom.co.nz/ideasroom/lessons-from-our-covid-tracing-app [accessed 27/08/2021].

Chen, J., & See, K. C. (2020). Artificial intelligence for COVID-19: Rapid review. *Journal of Medical Internet Research, 22*(10), e21476.

Chen, Z., Liu, Z., Ng, K. L., Yu, H., Liu, Y., & Yang, Q. (2020). A Gamified Research Tool for Incentive Mechanism Design in Federated Learning. In Yang, Q., Fan, L., Yu, H. (Eds.), *Federated Learning* (pp. 168–175). Springer, Cham.

Chirumamilla, A., & Sindre, G. (2021). E-exams in Norwegian higher education: Vendors and managers views on requirements in a digital ecosystem perspective. *Computers & Education, 172,* 104263.

Cho, J. K., Zafar, H. M., & Cook, T. S. (2020). Use of an online crowdsourcing platform to assess patient comprehension of radiology reports and colloquialisms. *American Journal of Roentgenology, 214*(6), 1316–1320.

Chou, Y. K. (2019). *Actionable Gamification: Beyond Points, Badges, and Leaderboards.* Birmingham, UK: Packt Publishing.

Choudrie, J., Banerjee, S., Kotecha, K., Walambe, R., Karende, H., & Ameta, J. (2021). Machine learning techniques and older adults processing of online information and misinformation: A covid 19 study. *Computers in Human Behavior, 119,* 106716.

Chrzan, R., Bociąga-Jasik, M., Bryll, A., Grochowska, A., & Popiela, T. (2021). Differences among COVID-19, Bronchopneumonia and Atypical Pneumonia in Chest High Resolution Computed Tomography

Assessed by Artificial Intelligence Technology. *Journal of Personalized Medicine*, *11*(5), 391.

Chung, A. E., Skinner, A. C., Hasty, S. E., & Perrin, E. M. (2017). Tweeting to health: A novel mHealth intervention using Fitbits and Twitter to foster healthy lifestyles. *Clinical Pediatrics*, *56*(1), 26–32.

Cichos, F., Gustavsson, K., Mehlig, B., & Volpe, G. (2020). Machine learning for active matter. *Nature Machine Intelligence*, *2*, 94–103.

Cincinnati Chindren's. (August 5, 2021). *Feeling Anxious About Our Troubled Times? This App May Help.* Retrieved from https://www.cinc innatichildrens.org/news/release/2020/covid-anxiety-app [accessed 31/08/2021].

Clare, C. A. (2021). Telehealth and the digital divide as a social determinant of health during the COVID-19 pandemic. *Network Modeling Analysis in Health Informatics and Bioinformatics*, *10*, 26.

Colizza, V., Grill, E., Mikolajczyk, R., Cattuto, C., Kucharski, A., Riley, S., ... & Fraser, C. (2021). Time to evaluate COVID-19 contact-tracing apps. *Nature Medicine*, *27*, 361–362.

Confalonieri, R., Weyde, T., Besold, T. R., & del Prado Martín, F. M. (2021). Using ontologies to enhance human understandability of global post-hoc explanations of black-box models. *Artificial Intelligence*, *296*, 103471.

Contreras-Espinosa, R. S., & Blanco, A. (2021). A literature review of e-government services with gamification elements. *International Journal of Public Administration*. In Press.

Coombs, C. (2020). Will COVID-19 be the tipping point for the intelligent automation of work? A review of the debate and implications for research. *International Journal of Information Management*, *55*, 102182.

Cope, B., Kalantzis, M., & Searsmith, D. (2020). Artificial intelligence for education: Knowledge and its assessment in AI-enabled learning ecologies. *Educational Philosophy and Theory*. In Press.

Cortés, U., Cortés, A., Garcia-Gasulla, D., Pérez-Arnal, R., Álvarez-Napagao, S., & Àlvarez, E. (2021). The ethical use of high-performance computing and artificial intelligence: Fighting COVID-19 at Barcelona Supercomputing Center. *AI and Ethics*. In Press.

Cossio, M., & Gilardino, R. E. (2021). Would the use of artificial intelligence in COVID-19 patient management add value to the healthcare system? *Frontiers in Medicine, 8*, 619202.

Covid19People. (2020). *Câmara Municipal de Câmara de Lobos.* Retrieved from https://pt.covid19people.help/issues/41/ [accessed 08/10/2021].

Cuevas-Lara, C., Izquierdo, M., de Asteasu, M. L. S., Ramírez-Vélez, R., Zambom-Ferraresi, F., Zambom-Ferraresi, F., & Martínez-Velilla, N. (2021). Impact of game-based interventions on health-related outcomes in hospitalized older patients: A systematic review. *Journal of the American Medical Directors Association, 22*(2), 364–371.

Dagliati, A., Malovini, A., Tibollo, V., & Bellazzi, R. (2021). Health informatics and EHR to support clinical research in the COVID-19 pandemic: An overview. *Briefings in Bioinformatics, 22*(2), 812–822.

De Freitas, M. (April 01, 2021). *uMore, the AI-powered mental wellbeing tracker, becomes the first UAE based start-up accepted to TheVentureCity.* uMore. Retrieved from https://umore.app/2021/04/01/umore-press-rele ase-umore-the-ai-powered-mental-wellbeing-tracker-becomes-the-first-uae-based-start-up-accepted-to-theventurecity/ [accessed 07/09/2021].

Delijewski, M., & Haneczok, J. (2021). AI drug discovery screening for COVID-19 reveals zafirlukast as a repurposing candidate. *Medicine in Drug Discovery, 9*, 100077.

Devine, D., Gaskell, J., Jennings, W., & Stoker, G. (2021). Trust and the coronavirus pandemic: What are the consequences of and for trust? An early review of the literature. *Political Studies Review, 19*(2), 274–285.

Dickinson, M. [@medickinson]. (April 8, 2021). *Who else has a swirly award for scanning in using NZ COVID Tracer? Today's update to the app includes this* [Tweet] [Image attached]. Twitter. https://twitter.com/ medickinson/status/1379917735837069312 [accessed 27/08/2021].

Dorr, F., Chaves, H., Serra, M. M., Ramirez, A., Costa, M. E., Seia, J., ... & Barmaimon, G. (2020). COVID-19 pneumonia accurately detected on chest radiographs with artificial intelligence. *Intelligence-Based Medicine, 3–4*, 100014.

Dotolo, S., Marabotti, A., Facchiano, A., & Tagliaferri, R. (2021). A review on drug repurposing applicable to COVID-19. *Briefings in Bioinformatics, 22*(2), 726–741.

Dou, Q., So, T. Y., Jiang, M., Liu, Q., Vardhanabhuti, V., Kaissis, G., ... & Heng, P. A. (2021). Federated deep learning for detecting COVID-19 lung abnormalities in CT: A privacy-preserving multinational validation study. *NPJ Digital Medicine, 4,* 60.

Dron, L., Dillman, A., Zoratti, M. J., Haggstrom, J., Mills, E. J., & Park, J. J. (2021). Clinical trial data sharing for COVID-19–related research. *Journal of Medical Internet Research, 23*(3), e26718.

Ekong, I., Chukwu, E., & Chukwu, M. (2020). COVID-19 mobile positioning data contact tracing and patient privacy regulations: Exploratory search of global response strategies and the use of digital tools in Nigeria. *JMIR mHealth and uHealth, 8*(4), e19139.

El-Haddadeh, R., Fadlalla, A., & Hindi, N. M. (2021). Is there a place for responsible artificial intelligence in pandemics? A tale of two countries. *Information Systems Frontiers.* In Press.

Elhajjar, S., Karam, S., & Borna, S. (2021). Artificial intelligence in marketing education programs. *Marketing Education Review, 31*(1), 2–13.

ELSA Speak. (n.d.). *FAQs.* Retrieved from https://elsaspeak.com/faqs [accessed 07/09/2021].

ELSA Speak. (March 19, 2020a). *ELSA Provides Free Access for K-12 Students Around the World.* Retrieved from https://blog.elsaspeak.com/en/elsa-provides-free-access-for-k-12-students-around-the-world/ [accessed 07/09/2021].

ELSA Speak. (March 31, 2020b). *ELSA Student Ambassador Program.* Medium. Retrieved from https://medium.com/elsa-speak/elsa-student-ambassador-program-2dd0150a7a81 [accessed 07/09/2021].

ELSA Speak. (28 October 2020c). *ELSA Speak app now available in 9 different languages (with the latest addition, Korean).* Retrieved from https://blog.elsaspeak.com/en/elsa-speak-app-now-available-in-9-different-languages-with-the-latest-addition-korean/ [accessed 11/09/2021].

Epstein, S. (June 23, 2020). *As the world stopped, these companies thrived under lockdown.* Wired. Retrieved from https://www.wired.co.uk/article/businesses-recover-coronavirus [accessed 11/09/2021].

Eruchalu, C. N., Pichardo, M. S., Bharadwaj, M., Rodriguez, C. B., Rodriguez, J. A., Bergmark, R. W., ... & Ortega, G. (2021). The expanding digital divide: Digital health access inequities during the COVID-19 pandemic in New York City. *Journal of Urban Health, 98*(2), 183–186.

Facebook. (May 12, 2020). *Using AI to detect COVID-19 misinformation and exploitative content*. Facebook AI. Retrieved from https://ai.faceb ook.com/blog/using-ai-to-detect-covid-19-misinformation-and-exploitat ive-content/ [accessed 08/25/2021].

Facebook. (April 15, 2021). *How maps built with Facebook AI can help with COVID-19 vaccine delivery*. Facebook AI. Retrieved from https:// ai.facebook.com/blog/how-maps-built-with-facebook-ai-can-help-with-covid-19-vaccine-delivery/ [accessed 08/25/2021].

Fahey, R. A., & Hino, A. (2020). COVID-19, digital privacy, and the social limits on data-focused public health responses. *International Journal of Information Management, 55*, 102181.

Feng, W., Tu, R., & Hsieh, P. (2020). Can gamification increases consumers' engagement in fitness apps? The moderating role of commensurability of the game elements. *Journal of Retailing and Consumer Services, 57*, 102229.

Fitbit. (2021). Retrieved from https://www.fitbit.com/global/us/home [accessed 09/09/2021].

Fitbod. (2021). *Our COVID-19 continued support*. Retrieved from https:// fitbod.me/covid-19-support/ [accessed 01/09/2021].

Fletcher, G., & Griffiths, M. (2020). Digital transformation during a lockdown. *International Journal of Information Management, 55*, 102185.

Flint, S. W., Piotrkowicz, A., & Watts, K. (2021). Use of Artificial Intelligence to understand adults' thoughts and behaviours relating to COVID-19. *Perspectives in Public Health*. In Press.

Fontana, M. T. (2020). Gamification of ChemDraw during the COVID-19 pandemic: Investigating how a serious, educational-game tournament (molecule madness) impacts student wellness and organic chemistry skills while distance learning. *Journal of Chemical Education, 97*(9), 3358–3368.

Fosso Wamba, S., Epie Bawack, R., Guthrie, C., Queiroz, M. M., & André Carillo, K. D. (2021). Are we preparing for a good AI society? A bibliometric review and research agenda. *Technological Forecasting and Social Change, 164*, 120482.

GamaLearn. (2021). *SwiftAssess AI Proctor*. Retrieved from https://swiftass ess.com/features/security/ai-proctor [accessed 30/08/2021].

Garvan Institute. (2021). *DreamLab*. Retrieved from https://www.garvan. org.au/support-us/dreamlab [accessed 07/09/2021].

Gasser, U., Ienca, M., Scheibner, J., Sleigh, J., & Vayena, E. (2020). Digital tools against COVID-19: Taxonomy, ethical challenges, and navigation aid. *The Lancet Digital Health*, 2(8), e425–e434.

Gibbon, A. (October 07, 2020). *How ex-Careem senior exec is driving home mental health message*. Arabian Business. Retrieved from https:// www.arabianbusiness.com/wellness/452609-how-ex-careem-senior-exec-is-driving-home-mental-health-message [accessed 07/09/2021].

Gilchrist, K. (October 15, 2020). *How this Vietnamese entrepreneur won Google's backing for her A.I. app*. CNBC. Retrieved from https://www. cnbc.com/2020/10/15/how-artificial-intelligence-app-elsa-founder-won-googles-investment.html [accessed 07/09/2021].

Goethe, O. (2020). Gamification for Good: Addressing Dark Patterns in Gamified UX Design. In: Dillon, R. (Ed.), *The Digital Gaming Handbook* (pp. 53–62). Bocaratón, FL: CRC Press.

Golden, E. A., Zweig, M., Danieletto, M., Landell, K., Nadkarni, G., Bottinger, E., ... & Charney, D. S. (2021). A resilience-building app to support the mental health of health care workers in the COVID-19 era: Design process, distribution, and evaluation. *JMIR Formative Research*, 5(5), e26590.

Golding, J. (February 25, 2021). *Cognita launches largest ever school group roll-out of AI*. IE Today. Retrieved from https://ie-today.co.uk/news/ cognita-launches-largest-ever-school-group-roll-out-of-ai/ [accesed 08/ 10/2021].

Goswami, U., Black, A., Krohn, B., Meyers, W., & Iber, C. (2019). Smartphone-based delivery of oropharyngeal exercises for treatment of snoring: A randomized controlled trial. *Sleep and Breathing*, 23, 243–250.

GOV.UK. (25 March 2020). *Government launches Coronavirus Information Service on WhatsApp*. Government of United Kingdom. Retrieved from https://www.gov.uk/government/news/government-launches-coronavirus-information-service-on-whatsapp [accessed 31/08/2021].

GOV.UK. (28 June 2021). *Freedom of Information request on systems used to support the proactive vigilance of the COVID-19 vaccination*

programme (FOI 21/512). Retrieved from https://www.gov.uk/governm
ent/publications/freedom-of-information-responses-from-the-mhra-
week-commencing-24-may-2021/freedom-of-information-request-on-
systems-used-to-support-the-proactive-vigilance-of-the-covid-19-vacc
ination-programme-foi-21512 [accessed 08/09/2021].

Government of India. (2021). *IndiaFightsCorona COVID-19*. MyGov.
Retrieved from https://www.mygov.in/covid-19/ [accessed 31/08/2021].

Gradescope. (13 March 2020). *Recent updates to help with urgent remote
assessment needs (responding to COVID-19)*. Medium. Retrieved from
https://blog.gradescope.com/recent-updates-to-help-with-urgent-remote-
assessment-needs-responding-to-covid-19-61dae0d57d4a [accessed 10/
09/2021].

Gradescope. (n.d.). *AI-assisted grading and answer groups*. Retrieved from
https://help.gradescope.com/article/mv8qkiux00-instructor-assignment-
ai-grading-answer-groups [accessed 10/09/2021].

Gran, A. B., Booth, P., & Bucher, T. (2021). To be or not to be algorithm
aware: A question of a new digital divide? *Information, Communication
& Society*, 24(12), 1779–1796.

Guarino, S., Pierri, F., Di Giovanni, M., & Celestini, A. (2021). Information
disorders during the COVID-19 infodemic: The case of Italian Facebook.
Online Social Networks and Media, 22, 100124.

Guckian, J., Eveson, L., & May, H. (2020). The great escape? The rise of
the escape room in medical education. *Future Healthcare Journal*, 7(2),
112–115.

Guérard-Poirier, N., Beniey, M., Meloche-Dumas, L., Lebel-Guay, F.,
Misheva, B., Abbas, M., ... & Patocskai, E. (2020). An educational network
for surgical education supported by gamification elements: Protocol for
a randomized controlled trial. *JMIR Research Protocols*, 9(12), e21273.

Guthrie, C., Fosso-Wamba, S., & Arnaud, J. B. (2021). Online consumer
resilience during a pandemic: An exploratory study of e-commerce
behavior before, during and after a COVID-19 lockdown. *Journal of
Retailing and Consumer Services*, 61, 102570.

Haleem, A., Javaid, M., Singh, R. P., & Suman, R. (2021). Applications of
Artificial Intelligence (AI) for cardiology during COVID-19 pandemic.
Sustainable Operations and Computers, 2, 71–78.

Hall, S., & Border, S. (2020). Online neuroanatomy education and its role during the coronavirus disease 2019 (COVID-19) lockdown. *World Neurosurgery, 139*, 628.

Hallak, J. A., Scanzera, A. C., Azar, D. T., & Chan, R. P. (2020). Artificial intelligence in ophthalmology during COVID-19 and in the post COVID-19 era. *Current Opinion in Ophthalmology, 31*(5), 447–453.

Hamari, J., & Koivisto, J. (2015). "Working out for likes": An empirical study on social influence in exercise gamification. *Computers in Human Behavior, 50*, 333–347.

Hao, K. (March 11, 2019). *A little-known AI method can train on your health data without threatening your privacy*. MIT Technology Review. Retrieved from https://www.technologyreview.com/2019/03/11/136710/a-little-known-ai-method-can-train-on-your-health-data-without-threatening-your-privacy/ [accessed 10/08/2020].

Hassan, L., & Hamari, J. (2020). Gameful civic engagement: A review of the literature on gamification of e-participation. *Government Information Quarterly, 37*(3), 101461.

Hatmal, M. M. M. M., Al-Hatamleh, M. A., Olaimat, A. N., Hatmal, M., Alhaj-Qasem, D. M., Olaimat, T. M., & Mohamud, R. (2021). Side effects and perceptions following COVID-19 vaccination in Jordan: A randomized, cross-sectional study implementing machine learning for predicting severity of side effects. *Vaccines, 9*(6), 556.

Hazell, W. (February 12, 2020). *Coronavirus: English-language schools in Hong Kong and China use AI to teach students remotely*. i News. Retrieved from https://inews.co.uk/news/education/schools-hong-kong-china-closed-coronavirus-ai-397175 [accessed 11/09/2021].

He, Q., Du, F., & Simonse, L. W. (2021). A patient journey map to improve the home isolation experience of persons with mild COVID-19: Design research for service touchpoints of artificial intelligence in eHealth. *JMIR Medical Informatics, 9*(4), e23238.

Hedlund, J., Eklund, A., & Lundström, C. (2020). Key insights in the AIDA community policy on sharing of clinical imaging data for research in Sweden. *Scientific Data, 7*, 331.

Heilweil, R. (January 28, 2020). *How AI is battling the coronavirus outbreak*. Vox. Retrieved from https://www.vox.com/recode/2020/1/28/21110902/artificial-intelligence-ai-coronavirus-wuhan [accessed 31/08/2021].

Heneghan, C. (August 19, 2020). *Early Findings from Fitbit COVID-19 Study Suggest Fitbit Devices Can Identify Signs of Disease at Its Earliest Stages*. Fitbit. Retrieved from https://blog.fitbit.com/early-findings-covid-19-study/ [accessed 09/09/2021].

Ho, I. M. K., Cheong, K. Y., & Weldon, A. (2021). Predicting student satisfaction of emergency remote learning in higher education during COVID-19 using machine learning techniques. *PLoS One, 16*(4), e0249423.

Hoffman, D. A. (2020). Increasing access to care: Telehealth during COVID-19. *Journal of Law and the Biosciences, 7*(1), lsaa043.

Hsia, B. C., Singh, A. K., Njeze, O., Cosar, E., Mowrey, W. B., Feldman, J., ... & Jariwala, S. P. (2020). Developing and evaluating ASTHMAXcel adventures: A novel gamified mobile application for pediatric patients with asthma. *Annals of Allergy, Asthma & Immunology, 125*(5), 581–588.

Huang, C. K., Chen, C. D., & Liu, Y. T. (2019). To stay or not to stay? Discontinuance intention of gamification apps. *Information Technology & People, 32*(6), 1423–1445.

Huang, D. H., & Chueh, H. E. (2021). Chatbot usage intention analysis: Veterinary consultation. *Journal of Innovation & Knowledge, 6*(3), 135–144.

Hung, M., Lauren, E., Hon, E. S., Birmingham, W. C., Xu, J., Su, S., ... & Lipsky, M. S. (2020). Social network analysis of COVID-19 sentiments: Application of artificial intelligence. *Journal of Medical Internet Research, 22*(8), e22590.

Huseynov, F. (2020). Gamification in E-Commerce: Enhancing Digital Customer Engagement Through Game Elements. In K. Sandhu (Ed.), *Digital Innovations for Customer Engagement, Management, and Organizational Improvement* (pp. 144–161). Hershey, PA: IGI Global.

IBM. (n.d.). *Watson*. Retrieved from https://www.ibm.com/watson [accessed 30/08/2021].

Ienca, M., & Vayena, E. (2020). On the responsible use of digital data to tackle the COVID-19 pandemic. *Nature Medicine, 26*(4), 463–464.

Iivari, N., Sharma, S., & Ventä-Olkkonen, L. (2020). Digital transformation of everyday life-How COVID-19 pandemic transformed the basic education of the young generation and why information management research should care? *International Journal of Information Management*, *55*, 102183.

Inkster, B., Sarda, S., & Subramanian, V. (2018). An empathy-driven, conversational artificial intelligence agent (Wysa) for digital mental well-being: Real-world data evaluation mixed-methods study. *JMIR mHealth and uHealth*, *6*(11), e12106.

Ishmaev, G., Dennis, M., & van den Hoven, M. J. (2021). Ethics in the COVID-19 pandemic: Myths, false dilemmas, and moral overload. *Ethics and Information Technology*, *23*(1), S19–S34.

Jadczyk, T., Wojakowski, W., Tendera, M., Henry, T. D., Egnaczyk, G., & Shreenivas, S. (2021). Artificial intelligence can improve patient management at the time of a pandemic: The role of voice technology. *Journal of Medical Internet Research*, *23*(5), e22959.

Jena, P. K. (2020). Impact of Covid-19 on higher education in India. *International Journal of Advanced Education and Research (IJAER)*, *5*(3), 77–81.

Jiao, Z., Choi, J. W., Halsey, K., Tran, T. M. L., Hsieh, B., Wang, D., ... & Bai, H. X. (2021). Prognostication of patients with COVID-19 using artificial intelligence based on chest x-rays and clinical data: A retrospective study. *The Lancet Digital Health*, *3*(5), e286–e294.

Jiménez-Luna, J., Grisoni, F., Weskamp, N., & Schneider, G. (2021). Artificial intelligence in drug discovery: Recent advances and future perspectives. *Expert Opinion on Drug Discovery*, *16*(9), 949–959.

Jiwani, R., Dennis, B., Bess, C., Monk, S., Meyer, K., Wang, J., & Espinoza, S. (2021). Assessing acceptability and patient experience of a behavioral lifestyle intervention using fitbit technology in older adults to manage type 2 diabetes amid COVID-19 pandemic: A focus group study. *Geriatric Nursing*, *42*(1), 57–64.

Joffe, A. R. (2021). COVID-19: Rethinking the lockdown groupthink. *Frontiers in Public Health*, *9*, 625778.

Kabudi, T., Pappas, I., & Olsen, D. H. (2021). AI-enabled adaptive learning systems: A systematic mapping of the literature. *Computers and Education: Artificial Intelligence*, *2*, 100017.

Kahn, J. (November 5, 2020). *U.K. to use A.I. to spot dangerous side effects in the millions of COVID-19 vaccinations it will deliver*. Fortune.

Retrieved from https://fortune.com/2020/11/05/u-k-a-i-covid-19-vacci nations-side-effects/ [accessed 08/09/2021].

Kahoot. (2021). *About us.* Retrieved from https://kahoot.com/company/ [accessed 08/09/2021].

Kalleny, N. K. (2020). Advantages of Kahoot! Game-based formative assessments along with methods of its use and application during the COVID-19 Pandemic in various live learning sessions. *Journal of Microscopy and Ultrastructure, 8*(4), 175.

Kalogiannakis, M., Papadakis, S., & Zourmpakis, A. I. (2021). Gamification in science education. A systematic review of the literature. *Education Sciences, 11*(1), 22.

Kamboj, S., Rana, S., & Drave, V. A. (2020). Factors driving consumer engagement and intentions with gamification of mobile apps. *Journal of Electronic Commerce in Organizations (JECO), 18*(2), 17–35.

Kang, J., Diao, Z., & Zanini, M. T. (2021). Business-to-business marketing responses to COVID-19 crisis: A business process perspective. *Marketing Intelligence & Planning, 39*(3), 454–468.

Kankanamge, N., Yigitcanlar, T., Goonetilleke, A., & Kamruzzaman, M. (2020). How can gamification be incorporated into disaster emergency planning? A systematic review of the literature. *International Journal of Disaster Resilience in the Built Environment, 11*(4), 481–506.

Kannan, S., Subbaram, K., Ali, S., & Kannan, H. (2020). The role of artificial intelligence and machine learning techniques: Race for covid-19 vaccine. *Archives of Clinical Infectious Diseases, 15*(2), e103232.

Karaman, O., Alhudhaif, A., & Polat, K. (2021). Development of smart camera systems based on artificial intelligence network for social distance detection to fight against COVID-19. *Applied Soft Computing, 110*, 107610.

Kasperbauer, T. J. (2021). Conflicting roles for humans in learning health systems and AI-enabled healthcare. *Journal of Evaluation in Clinical Practice, 27*(3), 537–542.

Kaushal, K., Sarma, P., Rana, S. V., Medhi, B., & Naithani, M. (2020). Emerging role of artificial intelligence in therapeutics for COVID-19: A systematic review. *Journal of Biomolecular Structure and Dynamics.* In Press.

Kaushik, A. C., & Raj, U. (2020). AI-driven drug discovery: A boon against COVID-19? *AI Open*, *1*, 1–4.

Ke, Y. Y., Peng, T. T., Yeh, T. K., Huang, W. Z., Chang, S. E., Wu, S. H., ... & Chen, C. T. (2020). Artificial intelligence approach fighting COVID-19 with repurposing drugs. *Biomedical Journal*, *43*(4), 355–362.

Kecojevic, A., Basch, C. H., Sullivan, M., & Davi, N. K. (2020). The impact of the COVID-19 epidemic on mental health of undergraduate students in New Jersey, cross-sectional study. *PLoS One*, *15*(9), e0239696.

Khakpour, A., & Colomo-Palacios, R. (2021). Convergence of gamification and machine learning: A systematic literature review. *Technology, Knowledge and Learning*, *26*(3), 597–636.

Kharbat, F. F. F., & Daabes, A. S. A. (2021). E-proctored examinations during the COVID-19 pandemic: A close understanding. *Education and Information Technologies*, *26*, 6589–6605. In Press.

Kiliç, M. (2021). Ethico-Juridical Dimension of Artificial Intelligence Application in the Combat to Covid-19 Pandemics. In S. Bozqus Kahyaoglu (Ed.), *The Impact of Artificial Intelligence on Governance, Economics and Finance, Volume I* (pp. 299–317). Springer, Singapore.

Kim, S. Y., & Grady, C. (2020). Ethics in the time of COVID: What remains the same and what is different. *Neurology*, *94*(23), 1007–1008.

Klock, A. C. T., Gasparini, I., Pimenta, M. S., & Hamari, J. (2020). Tailored gamification: A review of literature. *International Journal of Human-Computer Studies*, *144*, 102495.

Klugar, M., Riad, A., Mekhemar, M., Conrad, J., Buchbender, M., Howaldt, H. P., & Attia, S. (2021). Side effects of mRNA-based and viral vector-based COVID-19 vaccines among German healthcare workers. *Biology*, *10*(8), 752.

Koivisto, J., & Hamari, J. (2019). The rise of motivational information systems: A review of gamification research. *International Journal of Information Management*, *45*, 191–210.

Kolanska, K., Chabbert-Buffet, N., Daraï, E., & Antoine, J. M. (2020). Artificial intelligence in medicine: A matter of joy or concern? *Journal of Gynecology Obstetrics and Human Reproduction*, *50*(1), 101962.

Kondylakis, H., Katehakis, D. G., Kouroubali, A., Logothetidis, F., Triantafyllidis, A., Kalamaras, I., ... & Tzovaras, D. (2020). COVID-19 mobile apps: A systematic review of the literature. *Journal of Medical Internet Research, 22*(12), e23170.

Konstantakopoulos, I. C., Barkan, A. R., He, S., Veeravalli, T., Liu, H., & Spanos, C. (2019). A deep learning and gamification approach to improving human-building interaction and energy efficiency in smart infrastructure. *Applied Energy, 237,* 810–821.

Krass, M., Henderson, P., Mello, M. M., Studdert, D. M., & Ho, D. E. (2021). How US law will evaluate artificial intelligence for covid-19. *BMJ, 372,* n234.

Kretchy, I. A., Asiedu-Danso, M., & Kretchy, J. P. (2021). Medication management and adherence during the COVID-19 pandemic: Perspectives and experiences from low-and middle-income countries. *Research in Social and Administrative Pharmacy, 17*(1), 2023–2026.

Kricka, L. J., Polevikov, S., Park, J. Y., Fortina, P., Bernardini, S., Satchkov, D., ... & Grishkov, M. (2020). Artificial intelligence-powered search tools and resources in the fight against COVID-19. *EJIFCC, 31*(2), 106–116.

Krishnamurthy, S. (2020). The future of business education: A commentary in the shadow of the Covid-19 pandemic. *Journal of Business Research, 117,* 1–5.

Kumar, R., & Veer, K. (2021). How artificial intelligence and internet of things can aid in the distribution of COVID-19 vaccines. *Diabetes & Metabolic Syndrome, 15*(3), 1049–1050.

Kumm, A. J., Viljoen, M., & de Vries, P. J. (2021). The digital divide in technologies for autism: Feasibility considerations for low-and middle-income countries. *Journal of Autism and Developmental Disorders.* In Press.

La Moncloa. (April 8, 2020). *The Government launches Hispabot-Covid19, a consultation channel on COVID-19 via WhatsApp.* Government of Spain. Retrieved from https://www.lamoncloa.gob.es/serviciosdeprensa/notasprensa/asuntos-economicos/Paginas/2020/080420-consulta.aspx [accessed 31/08/2021].

Lai, J., & Widmar, N. O. (2021). Revisiting the digital divide in the COVID- 19 era. *Applied Economic Perspectives and Policy, 43*(1), 458–464.

Lalmuanawma, S., Hussain, J., & Chhakchhuak, L. (2020). Applications of machine learning and artificial intelligence for Covid-19 (SARS-CoV-2) pandemic: A review. *Chaos, Solitons & Fractals, 139*, 110059.

Laponogov, I., Gonzalez, G., Shepherd, M., Qureshi, A., Veselkov, D., Charkoftaki, G., ... & Veselkov, K. (2021). Network machine learning maps phytochemically rich "Hyperfoods" to fight COVID-19. *Human Genomics, 15*, 1.

Larson, D. B., Magnus, D. C., Lungren, M. P., Shah, N. H., & Langlotz, C. P. (2020). Ethics of using and sharing clinical imaging data for artificial intelligence: A proposed framework. *Radiology, 295*(3), 675–682.

Larsson, S., & Heintz, F. (2020). Transparency in artificial intelligence. *Internet Policy Review, 9*(2), 1–16.

Lassau, N., Ammari, S., Chouzenoux, E., Gortais, H., Herent, P., Devilder, M., ... & Blum, M. G. (2021). Integrating deep learning CT-scan model, biological and clinical variables to predict severity of COVID-19 patients. *Nature Communications, 12*, 634.

Latif, S., Usman, M., Manzoor, S., Iqbal, W., Qadir, J., Tyson, G., ... & Crowcroft, J. (2020). Leveraging data science to combat covid-19: A comprehensive review. *IEEE Transactions on Artificial Intelligence, 1*(1), 85–103.

Lau, A. (2020). New technologies used in COVID-19 for business survival: Insights from the Hotel Sector in China. *Information Technology & Tourism, 22*(4), 497–504.

Lavecchia, A. (2019). Deep learning in drug discovery: Opportunities, challenges and future prospects. *Drug Discovery Today, 24*(10), 2017–2032.

Legido-Quigley, H., Asgari, N., Teo, Y. Y., Leung, G. M., Oshitani, H., Fukuda, K., ... & Heymann, D. (2020). Are high-performing health systems resilient against the COVID-19 epidemic? *The Lancet, 395*(10227), 848–850.

Leitão, R., Maguire, M., Turner, S., & Guimarães, L. (2021). A systematic evaluation of game elements effects on students' motivation. *Education and Information Technologies*. In Press.

Lenert, L., & McSwain, B. Y. (2020). Balancing health privacy, health information exchange, and research in the context of the

COVID-19 pandemic. *Journal of the American Medical Informatics Association, 27*(6), 963–966.

Lenovo. (August 18, 2021). *Lenovo Foundation Partners with Solve Education! to Support STEM Education through Gamification*. Lenovo StoryHub. Retrieved from https://news.lenovo.com/foundation-solve-education-to-support-stem-gamification/ [accessed 31/08/2021].

Leonardi, P. M. (2021). COVID-19 and the new technologies of organizing: Digital exhaust, digital footprints, and artificial intelligence in the wake of remote work. *Journal of Management Studies, 58*(1), 249–253.

Li, T., Sahu, A. K., Talwalkar, A., & Smith, V. (2020a). Federated learning: Challenges, methods, and future directions. *IEEE Signal Processing Magazine, 37*(3), 50–60.

Li, Y., Horowitz, M. A., Liu, J., Chew, A., Lan, H., Liu, Q., ... & Yang, C. (2020b). Individual-level fatality prediction of COVID-19 patients using AI methods. *Frontiers in Public Health, 8*, 587937.

Li, Y., Shang, K., Bian, W., He, L., Fan, Y., Ren, T., & Zhang, J. (2020c). Prediction of disease progression in patients with COVID-19 by artificial intelligence assisted lesion quantification. *Scientific Reports, 10*, 22083.

Liang, F. (2020). COVID-19 and health code: How digital platforms tackle the pandemic in China. *Social Media + Society, 6*(3), 1–4.

Lieberman, M. (March 3, 2020). *Coronavirus Prompting E-Learning Strategies*. Education Week. Retrieved from https://www.edweek.org/technology/coronavirus-prompting-e-learning-strategies/2020/03 [accessed 03/09/2021].

Lier, L. M., & Breuer, C. (2019). The motivating power of gamification: Does the inclusion of game elements increase the effectiveness of worksite health promotion programs? *International Journal of Workplace Health Management, 13*(1), 1–15.

Lin, L., & Hou, Z. (2020). Combat COVID-19 with artificial intelligence and big data. *Journal of Travel Medicine, 27*(5), taaa080.

Lin, X., & Kishore, R. (2021). Social media-enabled healthcare: A conceptual model of social media affordances, online social support, and health behaviors and outcomes. *Technological Forecasting and Social Change, 166*, 120574.

Linardatos, P., Papastefanopoulos, V., & Kotsiantis, S. (2021). Explainable AI: A review of machine learning interpretability methods. *Entropy*, *23*(1), 18.

Long, J. B., & Ehrenfeld, J. M. (2020). The role of augmented intelligence (AI) in detecting and preventing the spread of novel coronaviruses. *Journal of Medical Systems*, *44*, 59.

López-Belmonte, J., Segura-Robles, A., Fuentes-Cabrera, A., & Parra-González, M. E. (2020). Evaluating activation and absence of negative effect: Gamification and Escape Rooms for learning. *International Journal of Environmental Research and Public Health*, *17*, 2224.

López-Cabrera, J. D., Orozco-Morales, R., Portal-Diaz, J. A., Lovelle-Enríquez, O., & Pérez-Díaz, M. (2021). Current limitations to identify COVID-19 using artificial intelligence with chest X-ray imaging. *Health and Technology*, *11*, 411–424.

Luan, H., Geczy, P., Lai, H., Gobert, J., Yang, S. J., Ogata, H., ... & Tsai, C. C. (2020). Challenges and future directions of big data and artificial intelligence in education. *Frontiers in Psychology*, *11*, 580820.

Luengo-Oroz, M., Pham, K. H., Bullock, J., Kirkpatrick, R., Luccioni, A., Rubel, S., ... & Mariano, B. (2020). Artificial intelligence cooperation to support the global response to COVID-19. *Nature Machine Intelligence*, *2*(6), 295–297.

Lynley, M. (December 5, 2016). *CENTURY dives Deep to track student performance and help teachers build custom curriculum*. TechCrunch. Retrieved from https://techcrunch.com/2016/12/05/century-dives-deep-to-track-student-performance-and-help-teachers-build-custom-curriculum/ [accessed 11/09/2021].

Madani, Y., Erritali, M., & Bouikhalene, B. (2021). Using artificial intelligence techniques for detecting Covid-19 epidemic fake news in Moroccan tweets. *Results in Physics*, *25*, 104266.

Marabelli, M., Vaast, E., & Li, J. L. (2021). Preventing the digital scars of COVID-19. *European Journal of Information Systems*, *30*(2), 176–192.

Markus, A. F., Kors, J. A., & Rijnbeek, P. R. (2020). The role of explainability in creating trustworthy artificial intelligence for health care: A comprehensive survey of the terminology, design choices, and evaluation strategies. *Journal of Biomedical Informatics*, *113*, 103655.

Marques, G., Drissi, N., de la Torre Díez, I., de Abajo, B. S., & Ouhbi, S. (2021). Impact of COVID-19 on the psychological health of university students in Spain and their attitudes toward Mobile mental health solutions. *International Journal of Medical Informatics*, *147*, 104369.

Martín-Sómer, M., Moreira, J., & Casado, C. (2021). Use of Kahoot! to keep students' motivation during online classes in the lockdown period caused by Covid 19. *Education for Chemical Engineers*, *36*, 154–159.

Masuda, Y., Zimmermann, A., Viswanathan, M., Bass, M., Nakamura, O., & Yamamoto, S. (2021). Adaptive enterprise architecture for the digital healthcare industry: A digital platform for drug development. *Information*, *12*(2), 67.

Mavroeidi, A. G., Kitsiou, A., Kalloniatis, C., & Gritzalis, S. (2019). Gamification vs. privacy: Identifying and analysing the major concerns. *Future Internet*, *11*(3), 67.

Mbunge, E., Akinnuwesi, B., Fashoto, S. G., Metfula, A. S., & Mashwama, P. (2021). A critical review of emerging technologies for tackling COVID-19 pandemic. *Human Behavior and Emerging Technologies*, *3*(1), 25–39.

McCarthy, H., Potts, H., & Fisher, A. (2021). Physical activity behavior before, during, and after COVID-19 restrictions: Longitudinal smartphone-tracking study of adults in the United Kingdom. *Journal of Medical Internet Research*, *23*(2), e23701.

Mesgarpour, M., Abad, J. M. N., Alizadeh, R., Wongwises, S., Doranehgard, M. H., Ghaderi, S., & Karimi, N. (2021). Prediction of the spread of Corona-virus carrying droplets in a bus-A computational based artificial intelligence approach. *Journal of Hazardous Materials*, *413*(5), 125358.

Meske, C., Bunde, E., Schneider, J., & Gersch, M. (2020). Explainable artificial intelligence: Objectives, stakeholders, and future research opportunities. *Information Systems Management*. In Press.

Metabiota. (2020). Retrieved from https://metabiota.com [accessed 31/08/2021].

Mian, A., & Khan, S. (2020). Coronavirus: The spread of misinformation. *BMC Medicine*, *18*, 89.

Miller, T. (2019). Explanation in artificial intelligence: Insights from the social sciences. *Artificial Intelligence*, *267*, 1–38.

Ministry of Health of New Zealand. (2021). *Using the NZ COVID Tracer app*. Retrieved from https://www.health.govt.nz/our-work/diseases-and-conditions/covid-19-novel-coronavirus/covid-19-resources-and-tools/nz-covid-tracer-app [accessed 27/08/2021].

Mirchi, N., Ledwos, N., & Del Maestro, R. F. (2021). Intelligent tutoring systems: Re-envisioning surgical education in response to COVID-19. *Canadian Journal of Neurological Sciences, 48*(2), 198–200.

Mishra, A., Shukla, A., & Sharma, S. K. (2021). Psychological determinants of users' adoption and word-of-mouth recommendations of smart voice assistants. *International Journal of Information Management*, 102413. In Press.

MIT App Inventor. (2021). *About us*. Retrieved from https://appinventor.mit.edu/about-us [accessed 08/09/2021].

MIT Enterprise Forum. (n.d.). *Alumni Directori. uMore*. MIT Enterprise Forum Pan Arab. Retrieved from https://www.mitefarab.org/en/startup/1060/umore [accessed 07/09/2021].

MIT Solve. (2021). Retrieved from https://solve.mit.edu/drive-investments-to-solver-teams [accessed 11/09/2021].

Mitchell, R., Schuster, L., & Jin, H. S. (2020). Gamification and the impact of extrinsic motivation on needs satisfaction: Making work fun? *Journal of Business Research, 106*, 323–330.

Modgil, S., Gupta, S., Stekelorum, R., & Laguir, I. (2021). AI technologies and their impact on supply chain resilience during COVID-19. *International Journal of Physical Distribution & Logistics Management*. In Press.

Mohammad-Rahimi, H., Nadimi, M., Ghalyanchi-Langeroudi, A., Taheri, M., & Ghafouri-Fard, S. (2021). Application of machine learning in diagnosis of COVID-19 through X-ray and CT images: A scoping review. *Frontiers in Cardiovascular Medicine, 8*, 638011.

Mohanty, S., Rashid, M. H. A., Mridul, M., Mohanty, C., & Swayamsiddha, S. (2020). Application of artificial intelligence in COVID-19 drug repurposing. *Diabetes & Metabolic Syndrome: Clinical Research & Reviews, 14*, 1027–1031.

Mondal, B. (2020) Artificial Intelligence: State of the Art. In: Balas V., Kumar R., Srivastava R. (Eds.), *Recent Trends and Advances in Artificial*

Intelligence and Internet of Things. Intelligent Systems Reference Library, vol. 172 (pp. 389–425). Cham: Springer.

Mozur, P., Zhong, R., & Krolik, A. (March 1, 2020). *In Coronavirus Fight, China Gives Citizens a Color Code, With Red Flags*. The New York Times. Retrieved from https://www.nytimes.com/2020/03/01/business/china-coronavirus-surveillance.html [accessed 10/10/2021].

Mu, Y., & Aletras, N. (2020). Identifying Twitter users who repost unreliable news sources with linguistic information. *PeerJ Computer Science, 6*, e325.

Muflih, S., Abuhammad, S., Karasneh, R., Al-Azzam, S., Alzoubi, K. H., & Muflih, M. (2020). Online education for undergraduate health professional education during the COVID-19 pandemic: Attitudes, barriers, and ethical issues. *Research Square*. In Press.

Murphy, K., Di Ruggiero, E., Upshur, R., Willison, D. J., Malhotra, N., Cai, J. C., ... & Gibson, J. (2021). Artificial intelligence for good health: A scoping review of the ethics literature. *BMC Medical Ethics, 22*, 14.

Mushtaq, J., Pennella, R., Lavalle, S., Colarieti, A., Steidler, S., Martinenghi, C. M., ... & De Cobelli, F. (2021). Initial chest radiographs and artificial intelligence (AI) predict clinical outcomes in COVID-19 patients: Analysis of 697 Italian patients. *European Radiology, 31*(3), 1770–1779.

Naudé, W. (2020). Artificial intelligence vs COVID-19: Limitations, constraints and pitfalls. *AI & Society, 35*(3), 761–765.

Naudé, W. (2021). Artificial intelligence: Neither Utopian nor apocalyptic impacts soon. *Economics of Innovation and New Technology, 30*(1), 1–23.

Neri, E., Coppola, F., Miele, V., Bibbolino, C., & Grassi, R. (2020a). Artificial intelligence: Who is responsible for the diagnosis? *La Radiologia Medica, 125*, 517–521.

Neri, E., Miele, V., Coppola, F., & Grassi, R. (2020b). Use of CT and artificial intelligence in suspected or COVID-19 positive patients: Statement of the Italian Society of Medical and Interventional Radiology. *La Radiologia Medica, 125*(5), 505–508.

Nieto-Escamez, F. A., & Roldán-Tapia, M. D. (2021). Gamification as online teaching strategy during COVID-19: A mini-review. *Frontiers in Psychology, 12*, 648552.

Niiler, E. (January 25, 2020). *An AI Epidemiologist Sent the First Warnings of the Wuhan Virus*. Wired. Retrieved from https://www.wired.com/story/ai-epidemiologist-wuhan-public-health-warnings/ [accessed 08/25/2021].

Nuance. (June 04, 2020). *Nuance AI technology enables organizations to prioritize and protect seniors through voice*. Retrieved from https://news.nuance.com/2020-06-04-La-tecnologia-de-IA-de-Nuance-permite-a-las-organizaciones-priorizar-y-proteger-a-las-personas-mayores-a-tra ves-de-la-voz [accessed 08/09/2021].

O'Connell, A., Tomaselli, P. J., & Stobart-Gallagher, M. (2020). Effective use of virtual gamification during COVID-19 to deliver the OB-GYN core curriculum in an emergency medicine resident conference. *Cureus, 12*(6), e8397.

Osmanlliu, E., Rafie, E., Bédard, S., Paquette, J., Gore, G., & Pomey, M. P. (2021). Considerations for the design and implementation of COVID-19 contact tracing apps: Scoping review. *JMIR mHealth and uHealth, 9*(6), e27102.

Pan, P., Li, Y., Xiao, Y., Han, B., Su, L., Su, M., ... & Xie, L. (2020). Prognostic assessment of COVID-19 in the intensive care unit by machine learning methods: Model development and validation. *Journal of Medical Internet Research, 22*(11), e23128.

Park, J., Han, J., Kim, Y., & Rho, M. J. (2021). Development, acceptance, and concerns surrounding app-based services to overcome the COVID-19 outbreak in South Korea: Web-based survey study. *JMIR Medical Informatics, 9*(7), e29315.

Park, S., & Kim, S. (2021). Is sustainable online learning possible with gamification-the effect of gamified online learning on student learning. *Sustainability, 13*, 4267.

Payrovnaziri, S. N., Chen, Z., Rengifo-Moreno, P., Miller, T., Bian, J., Chen, J. H., ... & He, Z. (2020). Explainable artificial intelligence models using real-world electronic health record data: A systematic scoping review. *Journal of the American Medical Informatics Association, 27*(7), 1173–1185.

Petch, J., Di, S., & Nelson, W. (2021). Opening the black box: The promise and limitations of explainable machine learning in cardiology. *Canadian Journal of Cardiology*. In Press.

Phillips Jr., E. G., Nabhan, C., & Feinberg, B. A. (2019). The gamification of healthcare: Emergence of the digital practitioner? *The American Journal of Managed Care, 25*(1), 13–15.

Pickering, B. (2021). Trust, but verify: Informed consent, AI technologies, and public health emergencies. *Future Internet, 13*(5), 132.

Polito, G., & Temperini, M. (2021). A gamified web based system for computer programming learning. *Computers and Education: Artificial Intelligence, 2*, 100029.

Putz, L. M., Hofbauer, F., & Treiblmaier, H. (2020). Can gamification help to improve education? Findings from a longitudinal study. *Computers in Human Behavior, 110*, 106392.

Qian, F., & Zhang, A. (2021). The value of federated learning during and post-COVID-19. *International Journal for Quality in Health Care, 33*(1), mzab010.

Quinn, T. P., Senadeera, M., Jacobs, S., Coghlan, S., & Le, V. (2021). Trust and medical AI: The challenges we face and the expertise needed to overcome them. *Journal of the American Medical Informatics Association, 28*(4), 890–894.

Raab, M. H., Döbler, N. A., & Carbon, C. C. (2021). A game of Covid: Strategic thoughts about a ludified pandemic. *Frontiers in Psychology, 12*, 607309.

Raftopoulos, M. (2014). Towards gamification transparency: A conceptual framework for the development of responsible gamified enterprise systems. *Journal of Gaming & Virtual Worlds, 6*(2), 159–178.

Ramon-Cortes, C., Alvarez, P., Lordan, F., Alvarez, J., Ejarque, J., & Badia, R. M. (2021). A survey on the distributed computing stack. *Computer Science Review, 42*, 100422.

Ramsetty, A., & Adams, C. (2020). Impact of the digital divide in the age of COVID-19. *Journal of the American Medical Informatics Association, 27*(7), 1147–1148.

Raza, K. (2020). Artificial Intelligence Against COVID-19: A Meta-Analysis of Current Research. In Hassanien AE., Dey N., Elghamrawy S. (Eds.), *Big Data Analytics and Artificial Intelligence Against COVID-19: Innovation Vision and Approach* (pp. 165–176). Cham: Springer.

Razami, H. H., & Ibrahim, R. (2021). Distance education during COVID-19 pandemic: The perceptions and preference of university students in

Malaysia towards online learning. *International Journal of Advanced Computer Science and Applications*, *12*(4), 118–126.

Reyna-Figueroa, J., Bejarano-Juvera, A. A., Arce-Salinas, C. A., Martínez-Arredondo, H., & Lehmann-Mendoza, R. (2020). Missed opportunities in medical specialty education, apropos of influenza and COVID-19. *Gaceta Médica de México*, *156*, 321–327.

Rezaei, N., & Grandner, M. A. (2021). Changes in sleep duration, timing, and variability during the COVID-19 pandemic: Large-scale Fitbit data from 6 major US cities. *Sleep Health*, *7*(3), 303–313.

Rieke, N., Hancox, J., Li, W., Milletari, F., Roth, H. R., Albarqouni, S., ... & Cardoso, M. J. (2020). The future of digital health with federated learning. *NPJ Digital Medicine*, *3*, 119.

Romano, M., Díaz, P., & Aedo, I. (2021). Gamification-less: May gamification really foster civic participation? A controlled field experiment. *Journal of Ambient Intelligence and Humanized Computing*. In Press.

Roy, R., & Naidoo, V. (2021). Enhancing chatbot effectiveness: The role of anthropomorphic conversational styles and time orientation. *Journal of Business Research*, *126*, 23–34.

Ryan, M. (2020). In defence of digital contact-tracing: Human rights, South Korea and Covid-19. *International Journal of Pervasive Computing and Communications*, *16*(4), 383–407.

Ryan, M., & Stahl, B. C. (2021). Artificial intelligence ethics ethics guidelines for developers and users: Clarifying their content and normative implications. *Journal of Information, Communication and Ethics in Society*, *19*(1), 61–86.

Sadoughifar, R., Goldust, M., Abdshahzadeh, H., Abrishamchi, R., Rudnicka, L., Jafferany, M., & Gupta, M. (2020). Artificial intelligence in diagnosis and management of COVID-19 in dermatology. *Dermatologic Therapy*, *33*, e13794.

Saeed, B. Q., Al-Shahrabi, R., Alhaj, S. S., Alkokhardi, Z. M., & Adrees, A. O. (2021). Side effects and perceptions following Sinopharm COVID-19 vaccination. *International Journal of Infectious Diseases*, *111*(October), 219–226.

Saeed, S. A., & Masters, R. M. (2021). Disparities in health care and the digital divide. *Current Psychiatry Reports*, *23*, 61.

Sahin, M., & Yurdugül, H. (2020). Learners' needs in online learning environments and third generation learning management systems (LMS 3.0). *Technology, Knowledge and Learning*. In Press.

Salvatore, C., Interlenghi, M., Monti, C. B., Ippolito, D., Capra, D., Cozzi, A., ... & Sardanelli, F. (2021). Artificial intelligence applied to chest X-ray for differential diagnosis of COVID-19 pneumonia. *Diagnostics,* *11*, 530.

Schlegelmilch, B. B. (2020). Why business schools need radical innovations: Drivers and development trajectories. *Journal of Marketing Education*, *42*(2), 93–107.

Schöbel, S. M., Janson, A., & Söllner, M. (2020). Capturing the complexity of gamification elements: A holistic approach for analysing existing and deriving novel gamification designs. *European Journal of Information Systems*, *29*(6), 641–668.

Seixas, A. A., Olaye, I. M., Wall, S. P., & Dunn, P. (2021). Optimizing healthcare through digital health and wellness solutions to meet the needs of patients with chronic disease during the COVID-19 era. *Frontiers in Public Health*, *9*, 667654.

Sekalala, S., Dagron, S., Forman, L., & Meier, B. M. (2020). Analyzing the human rights impact of increased digital public health surveillance during the COVID-19 crisis. *Health and Human Rights*, *22*(2), 7–20.

Shachar, C., Gerke, S., & Adashi, E. Y. (2020). AI surveillance during pandemics: Ethical implementation imperatives. *Hastings Center Report*, *50*(3), 18–21.

Shahi, G. K., Dirkson, A., & Majchrzak, T. A. (2021). An exploratory study of COVID-19 misinformation on Twitter. *Online Social Networks and Media*, *22*, 100104.

Shaikh, F., Andersen, M. B., Sohail, M. R., Mulero, F., Awan, O., Dupont-Roettger, D., ... & Bisdas, S. (2021). Current landscape of imaging and the potential role for artificial intelligence in the management of covid-19. *Current Problems in Diagnostic Radiology*, *50*(3), 430–435.

Shareef, M. A., Kumar, V., Dwivedi, Y. K., Kumar, U., Akram, M. S., & Raman, R. (2021). A new health care system enabled by machine intelligence: Elderly people's trust or losing self control. *Technological Forecasting and Social Change*, *162*, 120334.

Sharma, T., & Bashir, M. (2020). Use of apps in the COVID-19 response and the loss of privacy protection. *Nature Medicine, 26*(8), 1165–1167.

Shek, D. T. L. (2021). COVID-19 and quality of life: Twelve reflections. *Applied Research Quality Life, 16*, 1–11.

Silverman, M., Sibbald, R., & Stranges, S. (2020). Ethics of COVID-19-related school closures. *Canadian Journal of Public Health, 111*(4), 462–465.

Singh, H. J. L., Couch, D., & Yap, K. (2020). Mobile health apps that help with COVID-19 management: Scoping review. *JMIR Nursing, 3*(1), e20596.

Sipior, J. C. (2020). Considerations for development and use of AI in response to COVID-19. *International Journal of Information Management, 55*, 102170.

Smirnov, I. (2020). Estimating educational outcomes from students' short texts on social media. *EPJ Data Science, 9*, 27.

Snyder, A. (May 4, 2021). *PRESS RELEASE: MIT Solve Announces Four New Solve Innovation Future Investments in Early-Stage Social Entrepreneurs*. MIT Solve. Retrieved from https://solve.mit.edu/artic les/press-release-mit-solve-announces-four-new-solve-innovation-future-investments-in-early-stage-social-entrepreneurs [accessed 11/09/2021].

Solve Education. (2021a). *About Solve Education!* Retrieved from https:// solveeducation.org/old-homepage/ [accessed 31/08/2021].

Solve Education. (n.d. -a). *Learnalytics*. Retrieved from https://learnalytics. solveeducation.org [accessed 31/08/03].

Solve Education. (n.d.-b). *Dawn of Civilization*. Retrieved from https://sol veeducation.org/game-for-charity [accessed 31/08/2021].

Southwell, B. G., Niederdeppe, J., Cappella, J. N., Gaysynsky, A., Kelley, D. E., Oh, A., ... & Chou, W. Y. S. (2019). Misinformation as a misunderstood challenge to public health. *American Journal of Preventive Medicine, 57*(2), 282–285.

Spanakis, P., Peckham, E., Mathers, A., Shiers, D., & Gilbody, S. (2021). The digital divide: Amplifying health inequalities for people with severe mental illness in the time of COVID-19. *The British Journal of Psychiatry, 219*(4), 529–531.

Spanellis, A., Dörfler, V., & MacBryde, J. (2020). Investigating the potential for using gamification to empower knowledge workers. *Expert Systems with Applications, 160*, 113694.

Subudhi, S., Verma, A., & Patel, A. B. (2020). Prognostic machine learning models for COVID- 19 to facilitate decision making. *International Journal of Clinical Practice, 74*(12), e13685.

Summers, R. M. (2021). Artificial Intelligence of COVID-19 imaging: A hammer in search of a nail. *Radiology, 298*(3), e169–e171.

Suppan, M., Gartner, B., Golay, E., Stuby, L., White, M., Cottet, P., ... & Suppan, L. (2020a). Teaching adequate prehospital use of personal protective equipment during the COVID-19 pandemic: Development of a gamified e-learning module. *JMIR Serious Games, 8*(2), e20173.

Suppan, L., Abbas, M., Stuby, L., Cottet, P., Larribau, R., Golay, E., ... & Suppan, M. (2020b). Effect of an E-learning module on personal protective equipment proficiency among prehospital personnel: Web-based randomized controlled trial. *Journal of Medical Internet Research, 22*(8), e21265.

Swacha, J. (2021). State of research on gamification in education: A bibliometric survey. *Education Sciences, 11*, 69.

Tan, D. Y., & Cheah, C. W. (2021). Developing a gamified AI-enabled online learning application to improve students' perception to university physics. *Computers and Education: Artificial Intelligence, 2*, 100032.

Tang, G., Westover, K., & Jiang, S. (2021). Contact tracing in healthcare settings during the COVID-19 pandemic using bluetooth low energy and Artificial Intelligence-A viewpoint. *Frontiers in Artificial Intelligence, 4*, 666599.

Tang, G., Yan, Y., Shen, C., Jia, X., Zinn, M., Trivedi, Z., ... & Jiang, S. (2020). Development of a real-time indoor location system using bluetooth low energy technology and deep learning to facilitate clinical applications. *Medical Physics, 47*(8), 3277–3285.

Tarik, A., Aissa, H., & Yousef, F. (2021). Artificial Intelligence and machine learning to predict student performance during the COVID-19. *Procedia Computer Science, 184*, 835–840.

Tayal, S., Rajagopal, K., & Mahajan, V. (2020). Gratification through gamification in COVID 19? A study of gamification in an online virtual community and intrinsic need satisfaction during the global crisis. *Psychology and Education Journal*, *57*(9), 7364–7373.

TheVentureCity. (May 21, 2021) *Tucuvi, uMore and Bfore.ai join the team!* Retrieved from https://theventure.city/blog/2021/05/21/tucuvi-before-ai-y-umore-se-unen-al-equipo/?lang=es [accessed 07/09/2021].

Thorpe, A. S., & Roper, S. (2019). The ethics of gamification in a marketing context. *Journal of Business Ethics*, *155*(2), 597–609.

Tep, S. P., Cachecho, M., & Jean-Bouchard, É. (2021). Innovation, Ethics, and Consumer Protection: The Context of Fintech Gamification in Quebec. In *Ubiquitous Technologies for Human Development and Knowledge Management* (pp. 208–224). Hershey, PA: IGI Global.

Torda, A. (2020). How COVID-19 has pushed us into a medical education revolution. *Internal Medicine Journal*, *50*(9), 1150–1153.

TorreJuana. (13 March 2020). *Carina: Free public service to inform about Coronavirus*. Retrieved from https://ost.torrejuana.es/corina-gratuita-servicio-publico-informar-coronavirus/ [accessed 31/08/2021].

Tran, O. (April 19, 2019). *Vu Van's Journey In Building ELSA Speak*. Vietcetera. Retrieved from https://vietcetera.com/en/vu-vans-journey-in-building-elsa-speak [accessed 07/09/2021].

Trinidad, M., Ruiz, M., & Calderón, A. (2021). A bibliometric analysis of gamification research. *IEEE Access*, *9*, 46505–46544.

Turale, S., Meechamnan, C., & Kunaviktikul, W. (2020). Challenging times: Ethics, nursing and the COVID- 19 pandemic. *International Nursing Review*, *67*(2), 164–167.

Twitter. (March 16, 2020). *Our use of automated technology*. Coronavirus: Staying safe and informed on Twitter. Retrieved from https://blog.twitter.com/en_us/topics/company/2020/covid-19#misleadi nginformationupdate [accessed 01/09/2021].

Tzachor, A., Whittlestone, J., & Sundaram, L. (2020). Artificial intelligence in a crisis needs ethics with urgency. *Nature Machine Intelligence*, *2*, 365–366.

UKTN. (June 23, 2021). *British AI edtech startup, founded by female barrister-turned-entrepreneur, just raised $6.5M*. Retrieved from https://www.uktech.news/news/british-ai-edtech-startup-century-tech-funding-20210623 [accessed 11/09/2021].

uMore. (2020a). Retrieved from https://umore.app [accessed 07/09/2021].

uMore. (2020b). *Our science*. Retrieved from https://umore.app/the-umore-science/ [accessed 07/09/2021].

uMore. (2020c). *About us*. Retrieved from https://umore.app/about-us/ [accessed 07/09/2021].

uMore. (2020d). *Behavioural science*. Retrieved from https://umore.app/how-we-use-behavioural-science-at-umore/ [accessed 07/09/2021].

UNESCO (2020). *COVID-19 Impact on Education*. Retrieved from https://en.unesco.org/covid19/educationresponse [accessed 31/08/2021].

Vaishya, R., Javaid, M., Khan, I. H., & Haleem, A. (2020). Artificial Intelligence (AI) applications for COVID-19 pandemic. *Diabetes & Metabolic Syndrome: Clinical Research & Reviews*, 14(4), 337–339.

van Assen, M., Lee, S. J., & De Cecco, C. N. (2020). Artificial intelligence from A to Z: from neural network to legal framework. *European Journal of Radiology*, *129*, 109083.

Van Jaarsveld, G. M. (2020). The effects of COVID-19 among the elderly population: A case for closing the digital divide. *Frontiers in Psychiatry*, *11*, 577427.

Veselkov, K. (April 06, 2020). *Corona-AI UK: Harnessing the power of AI and mobile supercomputing for drug repurposing and food tailoring in the fight against the coronavirus epidemic*. Vodafone. Retrieved from https://www.vodafone.com/what-we-do/services/apps/dreamlab/uk/news/corona-ai [accessed 07/09/2021].

Veselkov, K., Gonzalez, G., Aljifri, S., Galea, D., Mirnezami, R., Youssef, J., ... & Laponogov, I. (2019). HyperFoods: Machine intelligent mapping of cancer-beating molecules in foods. *Scientific Reports*, *9*, 9237.

Vodafone. (2020). *DreamLab facilitates Imperial College London's breakthrough in finding drugs and foods that could benefit people with COVID-19*. Retrieved from https://www.saladeprensa.vodafone.es/c/notas-prensa/np_avances_dreamlab/ [accessed 07/09/2021].

Vodafone. (2021). *Together, in the UK we can help fight COVID-19 while we sleep*. Retrieved from https://www.vodafone.com/vodafone-foundation/focus-areas/dreamlab-app/uk [accessed 07/09/2021].

Walmsley, J. (2021). Artificial intelligence and the value of transparency. *AI & Society*, *36*(2), 585–595.

Waltz, E. (2020). AI takes its best shot: What AI can-and can't-do in the race for a coronavirus vaccine-[Vaccine]. *IEEE Spectrum*, *57*(10), 24–67.

Watson, D. S., Krutzinna, J., Bruce, I. N., Griffiths, C. E., McInnes, I. B., Barnes, M. R., & Floridi, L. (2019). Clinical applications of machine learning algorithms: Beyond the black box. *BMJ, 364,* 1886.

Weil, T., & Murugesan, S. (2020). IT risk and resilience-cybersecurity response to COVID-19. *IEEE Computer Architecture Letters, 22*(03), 4–10.

WhatsApp. (2021). *The World Health Organization launches WHO Health Alert on WhatsApp.* Retrieved from https://www.whatsapp.com/coro navirus/who/?lang=en [accessed 31/08/2021].

Whittaker, L., Mulcahy, R., & Russell-Bennett, R. (2021). 'Go with the flow' for gamification and sustainability marketing. *International Journal of Information Management, 61,* 102305.

Willems, S. H., Rao, J., Bhambere, S., Patel, D., Biggins, Y., & Guite, J. W. (2021). Digital solutions to alleviate the burden on health systems during a public health care crisis: COVID-19 as an opportunity. *JMIR mHealth and uHealth, 9*(6), e25021.

Williams, S. N., Armitage, C. J., Tampe, T., & Dienes, K. (2021). Public attitudes towards COVID-19 contact tracing apps: A UK-based focus group study. *Health Expectations, 24*(2), 377–385.

World Health Organization. (11 March 2020). *WHO Director-General's opening remarks at the media briefing on COVID-19 – 11 March 2020.* Retrieved from https://www.who.int/director-general/speeches/detail/ who-director-general-s-opening-remarks-at-the-media-briefing-on-covid-19---11-march-2020 [accessed 14/09/2021].

Wysa. (n.d.). *Meet Wysa.* Retrieved from https://www.wysa.io/meet-wysa [accessed 31/08/2021].

Xi, N., & Hamari, J. (2020). Does gamification affect brand engagement and equity? A study in online brand communities. *Journal of Business Research, 109,* 449–460.

Xing, F., Peng, G., Zhang, B., Li, S., & Liang, X. (2021). Socio-technical barriers affecting large-scale deployment of AI-enabled wearable medical devices among the ageing population in China. *Technological Forecasting and Social Change, 166,* 120609.

Xu, D., Guo, Y., & Huang, M. (2021). Can Artificial Intelligence improve firms' competitiveness during the COVID-19 pandemic: International evidence. *Emerging Markets Finance and Trade, 57*(10), 2812–2825.

Yang, H., & Li, D. (2021a). Health management gamification: Understanding the effects of goal difficulty, achievement incentives, and social networks on performance. *Technological Forecasting and Social Change, 169*, 120839.

Yang, H., & Li, D. (2021b). Understanding the dark side of gamification health management: A stress perspective. *Information Processing & Management, 58*(5), 102649.

Yang, Y., & Koenigstorfer, J. (2020). Determinants of physical activity maintenance during the Covid-19 pandemic: A focus on fitness apps. *Translational Behavioral Medicine, 10*(4), 835–842.

Yaşar, Ş., Çolak, C., & Yoloğlu, S. (2021). Artificial Intelligence-based prediction of Covid-19 severity on the results of protein profiling. *Computer Methods and Programs in Biomedicine, 202*, 105996.

Yoon, S., Goh, H., Nadarajan, G. D., Sung, S., Teo, I., Lee, J., ... & Teo, T. L. (2021). Perceptions of mobile health apps and features to support psychosocial well-being among frontline health care workers involved in the COVID-19 pandemic response: Qualitative study. *Journal of Medical Internet Research, 23*(5), e26282.

Zain, N. H. M., Johari, S. N., Aziz, S. R. A., Teo, N. H. I., Ishak, N. H., & Othman, Z. (2021). Winning the needs of the Gen Z: Gamified health awareness campaign in defeating COVID-19 pandemic. *Procedia Computer Science, 179*, 974–981.

Zainuddin, Z., Chu, S. K. W., Shujahat, M., & Perera, C. J. (2020). The impact of gamification on learning and instruction: A systematic review of empirical evidence. *Educational Research Review, 30*, 100326.

Zarocostas, J. (2020). How to fight an infodemic. *The Lancet, 395*(10225), 676.

Zawacki-Richter, O., Marín, V. I., Bond, M., & Gouverneur, F. (2020). Systematic review of research on artificial intelligence applications in higher education-where are the educators? *International Journal of Educational Technology in Higher Education, 16*, 39.

Zhang, C., & Lu, Y. (2021). Study on Artificial Intelligence: The state of the art and future prospects. *Journal of Industrial Information Integration, 23*, 100224.

Zhang, D., Liu, X., Shao, M., Sun, Y., Lian, Q., & Zhang, H. (2021a). The value of artificial intelligence and imaging diagnosis in the fight against COVID-19. *Personal and Ubiquitous Computing*. In Press.

Zhang, K., & Aslan, A. B. (2021). AI technologies for education: Recent research & future directions. *Computers and Education: Artificial Intelligence*, 2, 100025.

Zhang, S., Huang, S., Liu, J., Dong, X., Meng, M., Chen, L., ... & Chen, D. (2021b). Identification and validation of prognostic factors in patients with COVID-19: A retrospective study based on artificial intelligence algorithms. *Journal of Intensive Medicine*, 1(2), 103–109.

Zhang, W., Zhou, T., Lu, Q., Wang, X., Zhu, C., Sun, H., ... & Wang, F. Y. (2021c). Dynamic fusion-based federated learning for COVID-19 detection. *IEEE Internet of Things Journal*, 8(21), 15884–15891.

Zhou, C., Xiu, H., Wang, Y., & Yu, X. (2021a). Characterizing the dissemination of misinformation on social media in health emergencies: An empirical study based on COVID-19. *Information Processing & Management*, 58(4), 102554.

Zhou, S. L., Jia, X., Skinner, S. P., Yang, W., & Claude, I. (2021b). Lessons on mobile apps for COVID-19 from China. *Journal of Safety Science and Resilience*, 2(2), 40–49.

Zhou, Y., Wang, F., Tang, J., Nussinov, R., & Cheng, F. (2020). Artificial intelligence in COVID-19 drug repurposing. *The Lancet Digital Health*, 2(12), e667–e676.

Zimmermann, B. M., Fiske, A., Prainsack, B., Hangel, N., McLennan, S., & Buyx, A. (2021). Early perceptions of COVID-19 contact tracing apps in German-speaking countries: Comparative mixed methods study. *Journal of Medical Internet Research*, 23(2), e25525.

www.ingramcontent.com/pod-product-compliance
Lightning Source LLC
Chambersburg PA
CBHW030246100426
42812CB00002B/335